MALE PRACTICE

How Doctors Manipulate Women

Robert S. Mendelsohn, M.D.

Contemporary Books, Inc.
Chicago

Library of Congress Cataloging in Publication Data

Mendelsohn, Robert S.
    Male practice.

    Bibliography: p.
    1. Gynecology—United States.   2. Obstetrics—United
States.   3. Sexism in Medicine—United States.
4. Iatrogenic diseases—United States.   5. Women's
health services—United States.   I. Title.   [DNLM:
1. Obstetrics.   2. Gynecology.   3. Medicine.   4. Women.
WP 100 M537m]
RG67.U6M46   618   80-68601
ISBN 0-8092-5974-5
ISBN 0-8092-5721-1(pbk.)

Published by Contemporary Books, Inc.
180 North Michigan Avenue, Chicago, Illinois 60601
Manufactured in the United States of America
Library of Congress Catalog Card Number: 80-68601
International Standard Book Number: 0-8092-5974-5
                                    0-8092-5721-1

Published simultaneously in Canada by
Beaverbooks, Ltd.
150 Lesmill Road
Don Mills, Ontario M3B 2T5
Canada

Contents

Acknowledgments

I'm grateful to the thousands of women I've encountered on radio or television and in my private practice whose provocative questions and revealing accounts of medical mayhem motivated me to write this book. Their sure instinct for truth and their critical appraisal of my views qualify them as the best faculty a lifelong student like me has ever had.

That role was shared by the media interviewers—print, audio, and video—and their associates, whose thoughtful probing has sharpened my positions and refined my verbal and written expressions. Even when I have been quoted out of context or freely paraphrased they have often managed to make my point more clearly than I did myself.

I'm also indebted to the many doctors, nurses, and dentists who have written me confessing that they have been "closet medical heretics," but now plan to assume a more activist role. Thanks to them, my writings, which began as a catharsis, have now evolved into a crusade. My gratitude for that support within my profession also extends to the medical students and their organizations across the country who have provided an appreciative forum for my heretical opinions.

Nor can I overlook the physicians in high places who have appeared with me on local and national media and public platforms. They have included the executive vice president of the American Medical Association, the president of the American College of Obstetrics and Gynecology, faculty members from Harvard and other prestigious medical schools, and the presidents or members of many local medical societies. Their determined defense of the indefensible has reinforced my determination to continue exposing medical practices that I abhor.

I'm also grateful to:

Phil Drotning, who gave wholeheartedly of his spirit as well as his outstanding professional writing skill to this book;

My daughters, Ruth and Sally, their husbands, Marty and David, and my grandchildren, Channa and Jonah (born Yom Kippur, 1980), whose examples in matters of health and otherwise I strive to follow;

Above all, my wife, who continues to provide the wisdom, stability, security, protection, and love that affords me the opportunity for thinking and the luxury of writing.

Robert S. Mendelsohn, M.D.

Introduction

If you read *Confessions of a Medical Heretic,* you already know that I despise the *institution* of Modern Medicine, which I have been battling quietly for nearly thirty years. In that book I tried to reveal the insidious and often lethal ritual of medical practice in the United States and to alert my readers to the ways in which today's doctors fail their patients and abuse the trust that is placed in them. When I had finished I thought, "That's that. I got it off my chest, and I'll never have to write a book again."

After *Confessions* was published, I discovered one of the side effects of authorship—a rash of invitations to appear on the lecture circuit and on radio and television shows. I toured the country for weeks, giving interviews and answering questions posed by studio audiences and listeners who called in on the phone. Often I found myself a dismayed but sympathetic listener as they related their own tragic experiences at the hands of doctors they thought they could trust. It took only a few sessions with Phil Donahue and other talk show hosts for me to realize that *Confessions* had merely exposed the tip of the iceberg as far as medical excesses, incompetence, and abuse are concerned.

Many of the programs on which I appeared were directed specifically toward women. Those audiences confirmed with stark and shocking clarity something I had long suspected, but had not really focused on before:

Although medical and surgical overkill are routinely inflicted on all Americans, its primary victims are women.

I noted a strong indication of this disparity in the statistical evidence I had gathered for *Confessions,* but mere numbers don't disclose the human aspects of any tragedy. The reality of medical abuse of women came pouring out of the talk show telephones in an endless stream of heartrending case histories. I heard first-person accounts of mistreatment, malpractice, death, and injury that put flesh on the statistical bones. In most instances the women I talked to were themselves the victims. In others, their lives had been shattered or diminished by the needless death or suffering of a husband or some other loved one.

These always plaintive, sometimes angry, and often desperate women represented the legion of women in the United States who are among the walking wounded—mentally, emotionally, physically disfigured by the very doctors they thought were on their side. I knew I could do little to help them, but perhaps I could help other women avoid a similar fate. That is why I had to write this book.

A final note: I titled this book *Male Practice* and deliberately use the masculine pronoun in reference to doctors because most American doctors are men. However, this doesn't imply that women physicians are absolved from the abuses I cite. Certainly they are better able to relate to female patients, and they are free of all of the chauvinistic garbage carried around by men. But female doctors *did* go to the same medical schools as male doctors. They *had* to employ the same artifices and devices to compete and survive. They *were* influenced by the same ridiculous and dangerous dogma. Consequently, most of them emerged from medical schools and hospital residencies brainwashed to practice medicine very much as though they were men.

MALE PRACTICE

1
"Trust Me, Dear."

Male chauvinism pervades American medicine from the doors of medical school to the slabs of the hospital morgue. Clearly, sexist behavior is at the heart of the medical abuse that women suffer. It is, however, compounded by the very fact that women visit doctors seven times as often as do men—with an attendant increase in risks.

That may sound contradictory if Modern Medicine has convinced you that regular visits to the doctor's office are vital way stations on the road to a long and rewarding life. Believe me, they're not. The door to the doctor's office ought to bear a surgeon general's warning that routine physical examinations are dangerous to your health. Why? Because doctors do not see themselves as guardians of health, and they have learned precious little about how to assure it. Instead, they are latter-day Don Quixotes, battling sometimes real but too often imaginary diseases. The disastrous difference is that doctors are not tilting at windmills. Rather, it is people who are damaged by their insistent search for dubious diseases to conquer.

There is no limit to the ingenuity of Modern Medicine in diagnosing diseases—or non-diseases—that it can treat. Doctors have been taught to seek, find, and treat illness, not to help you maintain good health. Consequently, when you visit your doctor for a routine physical checkup, it doesn't make much difference how healthy you are or how good you feel. Your naked and defenseless presence in his examining room is an open invitation to the doctor to declare that you are sick. By the time you've been psychologically traumatized by his questioning, poking, prodding, and testing, and you have taken a few of the pills he prescribes for the innocuous aberrances he has found, you may very well experience so many side effects that you really *are* sick.

Let's hypothesize a case history, just to see what can happen.

Mary is a recently married woman who is in perfect health. She becomes pregnant and, like most women, has been led to believe that she and her baby will be healthier if she makes a prenatal visit to her obstetrician once a month. He promptly begins treating her pregnancy as though it were a disease requiring radical medical intervention rather than a joyous, perfectly normal physiological event. Ultimately, after an exotic array of obstetrical wizardry, which makes the experience as difficult, dangerous, and distressing to the mother as possible, the doctor—not the mother—delivers the baby. By Caesarean section, no less, because the obstetrician is already late for a round of golf.

If Mary's baby survives the hazards of prenatal drugs and diets, amniocentesis, anesthesia, induced labor, and the infections rampant in the hospital nursery, the happy mother can take her child home from the hospital. If she's lucky, she may even be sent home with the right baby, but it will be hard for her to tell, for they've scarcely let her see the child during her hospital stay. Whether the baby is hers or not, however, Modern Medicine has a welcome new client for its services and wares.

Mary and her baby now begin a protracted series of ritual visits to the pediatrician. He'll advise unsound dietary practices in lieu of breast-feeding, administer dangerous inoculations, and solemnly collect statistics on length, weight, and when the baby rolls over, sits up, walks, talks, and stops wetting the bed. All of these data are entered into a neat little book, which makes a nice memento. They're also compared with a lot of data on pediatric progress that is recorded on the doctor's meaningless charts—which makes trouble. If Mary's baby fails to conform to the average height and weight, or to perform its gymnastics at precisely the right point in time, the pediatrician will seize the opportunity to launch the poor child on a lifetime of medical intervention. He probably won't tell Mary that the standard weight chart used by most doctors was drawn decades ago from a sample of 200 Irish kids in a Boston neighborhood and has little or no relevance to her child.

Mary, meanwhile, has been sold a bill of goods on the virtues of the annual Pap smear, an unnecessary and discredited ritual that keeps gynecologists busy and rich. If one of the results of these notoriously inaccurate tests looks even mildly suspicious, the gynecologist may talk her into having a hysterectomy, "just in case" cancer cells may be lurking about her uterus. While he's at it, he decides—without asking first—to take out the tubes and ovaries as well. This produces a probable disturbance of sexual function, creating business for the psychiatrists, to say nothing of the discomforts of premature menopause. But this is no problem for anyone but Mary, and perhaps her husband. The gynecologist puts her on a daily ration of estrogens to relieve the menopausal symptoms, and this keeps her coming back for checkups and refills that go on, although they shouldn't, for years and years.

Eventually, if Mary is really unlucky, she finds herself in the hands of a surgeon, facing the prospect of a radical mastectomy for cancer of the breast. She isn't told of the less radical, less disfiguring procedures that are available and produce equal or even better results. And you can bet that she isn't told that *it was the estrogens her gynecologist has been feeding her that produced the cancer in her breast.*

Mary's experience, though hypothetical, provides an unappetizing smorgasbord of the callous, indifferent, and dangerous interventions that Modern Medicine thrusts upon women. The greater tragedy is that they are inflicted on patients who don't know, or even suspect, that their own doctor is causing many of the ailments that he treats. Modern Medicine has surrounded itself with a mystique so intimidating that most patients accept their physician's orders, his potions, and even his surgery, without doubt or question. Theirs is not to reason why. Theirs is but to take the pills and die.

In the introduction to *Confessions of a Medical Heretic* I outlined the reasons for my lack of confidence in the institution of Modern Medicine. So that you'll know up front where I'm coming from when I discuss the medical abuse of women, let me restate those beliefs here.

I believe that the greatest danger to your health is the doctor who practices Modern Medicine.

I believe that Modern Medicine's treatments for disease are seldom effective and often more dangerous than the ailments they're employed to treat.

I believe that the dangers are compounded by the widespread use of dangerous procedures to treat *non-diseases,* procedures that produce *real* diseases that the doctor will then address with even more dangerous procedures in his efforts to repair the damage he has done.

I believe that Modern Medicine endangers its victims by attacking minor ailments with hazardous treatments that should only be used when the patient's life is at stake.

I believe that most doctors are the willing, if unwitting, tools of pharmaceutical manufacturers. Their patients become human guinea pigs for mass testing of drugs with dubious benefits and potentially lethal side effects that are unknown.

I believe that more than 90 percent of Modern Medicine could disappear from the face of the earth—doctors, hospitals, drugs, and equipment—and the health of the nation would immediately and dramatically improve.

As you might surmise, my heretical criticism of the institution of Modern Medicine—or the religion of Modern Medicine, as I prefer to think of it—often raises the hackles of medical professionals who read what I write or hear me speak. A typical comment goes something like this:

"I agree with some of what you say, Doctor, but you shouldn't generalize so much. You shouldn't talk in such absolute terms because it destroys your credibility."

I find it incredible that so many doctors who disagree violently with my views are so eager to enhance my credibility. But I know what they are trying to do. They are trying to win a dispensation that distinguishes them from the rest of the profession. I'm not buying that ploy. If I were to allow for the possibility that even one doctor may have escaped unscathed from the destructive influences of Modern Medicine, the game would be lost. Every doctor in the country would hasten to agree with me but claim exemption as a good guy and attribute the shenanigans to all of his peers.

I don't believe for a moment that all doctors, or even a majority of them, consciously attempt to mistreat, mislead, deceive, or cheat their patients. Some do, for in my profession, as in all others, there are idiots, crooks, incompetents, and scalawags. My criticism is directed toward the institution of medicine—the religion of medicine. Every patient is threatened by the subtle influence its traditions and teachings have on doctors who were brainwashed in medical school and then overwhelmed by peer pressure after they launched their medical careers.

In *Confessions of a Medical Heretic* I dealt with this concept in some depth, and I'm not going to repeat myself here. If those views intrigue you, read that book. The point is, and this is why I generalize, that *all* doctors are influenced, to varying degrees, by the dogma imposed on them in medical school. I'm concerned about that because I know that medical schools teach a great deal of professional misconduct, neatly cloaked in pious rhetoric. The character and behavior of the students are altered by it. You—the patient—pay the always costly and sometimes mortal price. That's why I am unwilling to let anyone in the medical profession, including myself, off the hook.

Doctors like to boast about the technical advances that have been made in medicine—the "miracle drugs," the exotic surgery, the sophisticated CAT-scanners, fetal monitors, EEG, EKG, and x-ray machines. But what do we have to show for the nation's $212 billion annual medical bill? What is the bottom line of all the years invested in medical education, the billions invested in hospitals and equipment, and the so-called progress represented by all of the marvelous machines?

Mortality rates are about the only measurement one can use to compare today's results with those of a century ago. If you make that comparison, excluding the lives saved by improved sanitation, better nutrition, and more sanitary living conditions that accompany an affluent society—plus a few major break-throughs in epidemiology, such as the conquest of malaria and typhus—the vaunted medical progress fades away. Americans aren't as healthy today as they were before all this new technology, pharmacology, and surgery appeared on the scene. Moreover, despite higher medical expenditures, more doctors, and more hospital beds—perhaps *because* of them—Americans aren't as healthy as residents of many other nations in the developed world!

Infant and maternal mortality rates offer startling evidence of this. The American College of Obstetrics and Gynecology (ACOG) is fond of claiming that its members deserve credit for the decline in infant and maternal death rates of the twentieth century. They don't tell you that much of this drop occurred during a time when most babies were delivered at home, with minimal obstetrical intervention, and that there has been little change in infant or maternal mortality rates since 1951, the year in which ACOG was formed. They also fail to tell you that infant mortality rates in the United States are almost double those of the Scandinavian countries and higher than those of fourteen other nations. You'll certainly never learn from your obstetrician that if you want to have your baby in the safest place you should go to Sweden, Holland, or Norway, or that you'd even be better off in Iceland or Taiwan!

What we have seen in Modern Medicine is not progress but

the *illusion* of progress. Repeatedly, one year's "progress" *causes* another year's ailments, for which new forms of interventionist "cures" will be developed. Thus, much of the so-called progress is nothing more than harmful intervention feeding on itself.

The question that worries me, and should worry you, won't be answered until we discover the long-term effects of all the radical pharmaceutical and surgical interventions of recent decades, much of it inflicted on women. There is already significant evidence that the highly toxic drugs that doctors have prescribed, the radical surgery that they have performed, and the needless x-rays that they have ordered may have killed more patients than they cured. But I'm convinced that this is only the beginning. It will be years before much of the latent damage that has already been done begins to appear.

During the two years that have elapsed since *Confessions of a Medical Heretic* was published, a number of potentially significant changes in recommended medical practice have been announced by some of the foremost medical organizations, and other hopeful signs have emerged. The following are examples.

The American Medical Association (AMA) abandoned its longtime advocacy of annual physical examinations, which I have long insisted create more ailments than they detect. It also revised its code of ethics to urge—*for the first time!*—that doctors stop covering up each other's mistakes and report instances of malpractice that they observe among their peers.

The American Cancer Society (ACS) reversed its position on the routine use of mammography examinations to detect breast cancer. This came in belated recognition of the fact that these x-ray examinations often lead to needless surgery and may cause more cancer than they detect. ACS also withdrew its recommendation of routine annual Pap smears except where justified by specific need.

The National Institutes of Health (NIH) shot down the long-held obstetrical concept that once a woman gives birth by Caesarean section, all subsequent babies must be delivered in the same hazardous way.

The U.S. Food and Drug Administration (FDA), after nearly twenty years of delay, announced that it would order the removal of some 3,000 drugs from the market. Why? Because, although Americans have spent billions of dollars on them, the manufacturers still haven't proved that they are effective.

Radio and television interviewers are fond of insisting that I take credit, because of the charges I made in *Confessions,* for bringing about these changes. It's tempting, because it would be nice to take some credit I don't deserve to make up for all of the undeserved criticism that I receive. But, before I do, I want to see whether the policies that their leaders are announcing are reflected in the ways that doctors behave. I'm dubious, because I have never known Modern Medicine voluntarily to give up any form of dangerous or unnecessary intervention unless it had a more dangerous and unnecessary procedure ready to take its place.

My suspicions were sharpened in the fall of 1980 when I participated in a debate with the incoming president of the ACOG. If I had been a little more naive, he might have softened me up because he was so very, very nice to me. He told the audience how useful it was to have someone within the medical profession who held up a mirror so doctors could look at themselves and mend their ways. Flattery was almost getting him somewhere until he went on to maintain that, indeed, obstetricians and gynecologists *had* mended their ways. Husbands, he said, were now routinely welcomed into hospital delivery rooms and even into the operating room when Caesarean sections were performed. Homelike hospital birthing rooms were popping up like daffodils. Obstetricians were encouraging breast-feeding.

The implication of all this was that my previous criticism, which he couldn't dispute, had done its work. Modern Medicine had reformed, and all of my old accusations were out of date. Obstetricians and gynecologists had heeded my complaints and didn't need my mirror any more, so I could put it away.

By the time the meeting ended, any temptation I may have had to claim credit for inducing changes in medical practice had faded away. It was obvious that the professed reforms were just so much window dressing. They would be used as a smoke screen to convince the clients of Modern Medicine that the mistreatment and malpractice were ancient history and that we had seen the dawn of a bright new day.

I won't deny that I am mildly encouraged by the changes that have been announced by the AMA, the ACS, the NIH, the ACOG, and the FDA. If those segments of the medical alphabet are serious about their new rules, there will be less chance that the rest of us will prematurely RIP. But rhetoric isn't reality. Until I see convincing, sustained evidence that doctors are practicing what their leaders are preaching, I'm not going to put my mirror away.

2

"It's a Good Thing You Came to See Me When You Did."

Women are the victims of so much dangerous and unnecessary medical and surgical intervention that watching what happens to them at the hands of their doctors makes me sick. Much of the time it also makes *them* sick.

Don't misunderstand me. I don't believe that very much of this medical abuse occurs because doctors are consciously greedy, or even inept. It happens because doctors haven't been taught to keep you healthy. They've been taught to believe that almost everyone is sick. Since your doctor is the sole arbiter of your physical condition, and because he *expects* you to be unhealthy, it is easy for him to find symptoms that will convince him, and help him convince you, that you really *are* sick.

Keep that in mind when your doctor tells you that it's a good thing you came to see him when you did. Is it a good thing for you or a good thing for him?

Those who face death sometimes view life with a clarity not given to those of us who have not lived out our years. In 1980, as he lay dying of cancer, an eminent seventy-one-year-old internist, Dr. Frederick Stenn, made his final assessment of Modern Medicine in a letter to the *New England Medical Journal.* It was published under the title, "Thoughts of a Dying Physician." This is what he said:

> Most physicians have lost the pearl that was once an intimate part of medicine—humanism. Machinery, efficiency, precision have driven from the heart warmth, compassion, sympathy and concern for the individual. Medicine is now an icy science. Its charm belongs to another age. The dying man can get little comfort from the mechanical doctor.

Dr. Stenn, whom I knew as a faculty member at the Northwestern University Medical School, had practiced in Chicago for forty-six years. He was recalling the era during which our grandparents and great-grandparents were growing up and the doctor's job was to make you well, not to make you sick. Medical practice was a labor-intensive profession, and most doctors didn't know a driver from a divot because they were on call twenty-four hours a day, seven days a week. The only time they saw a golf course was when one of their patients had a heart attack on the green.

Half a century ago doctors expected to make house calls when their patients were sick. They didn't tell mothers to bring their feverish babies to the office in order to save themselves a trip. They waited in the parlor for hours in order to be on hand for the blessed event, with no thought of inducing labor so that they could get home on time for dinner. They weren't there to intervene in the natural process of birth and to *deliver* the baby, but to *help the mother deliver it* in those rare instances when something went wrong.

In those days doctors knew their patients as human beings, not as scribbles on a chart. They knew whole families and even family trees. They didn't walk into the examining room on your sixth or eighth or tenth visit, pick up your file, and muse absentmindedly, "Let's see; I believe you've been here before."

Many doctors didn't even have an examining room. Their patients were greeted in a comfortable, reassuring office, not herded into cubicles to await their fate like so many defenseless sheep.

The family physician was willing to spend time with those who sought his help, listening to their woes, getting to know them, and providing comfort as well as advice. He cured a lot of ailments with doses of sympathy, kindness, reassurance, and plain old-fashioned common sense.

Doctors were trained—or taught themselves—to use their senses, their judgment, and even their intuition to diagnose their patients' ills. Using these priceless skills, most of them could make a clinical diagnosis that was more accurate than those arrived at today through batteries of often questionable computerized laboratory tests. Natural remedies weren't the butt of medical humor; they still had credibility, *and many of them really worked!* I guess the only survivor can be found in the Jewish branch of Modern Medicine—chicken soup!

Doctors were not yet the captives of the drug company detail men, so the toxic chemicals now sold by the ton were rarely used. Tests had not been substituted for wisdom, knowledge, and judgment, and they were seldom administered. Surgery, recognized as a dangerous treatment alternative, was something to be feared and avoided—the physician's last resort. X-rays weren't spreading cancer throughout the universe, and if you were sent to a hospital, you were probably on the verge of death.

One has to wonder why Modern Medicine is so proud that subtly, over half a century or so, highly structured medical education, technology, and specialty practice have changed all that. To the joy of doctors, who are now paid more for working less, and the sorrow of everyone else, medical practice has deliberately been dehumanized. It is no longer labor-intensive but expensively capital-intensive. The patient has become an object on the assembly line—or disassembly line—of a huge, overstaffed, well-oiled, impersonal machine.

More often than not, it is women who get caught in its cogs.

Unfortunately for its victims, the machine needs raw material to keep running. Modern Medicine is as concerned about that as General Motors, because when the assembly line isn't running it isn't paying for itself. The need to keep beds full and machines busy is at the top of the priority list of hospital administrators, well ahead of sanitation, safety, and medical care. At a retreat for the directors of a suburban hospital an executive conducted a seminar last year on "creative hospital marketing." He called it "a must in the highly competitive environment of health care institutions." It may not square with your perception of hospitals as caring nonprofit institutions, but he was simply pointing up the fact that the nation has too many hospitals and too many beds. It takes a lot of "creative marketing" to keep bodies in the beds.

That wouldn't be threatening if it were simply a matter of marketing strategies that kept one hospital filled at the expense of the others. Unfortunately, in most urban areas, there are also too many doctors. A piece of that creative marketing is an abundance of *creative diagnosis* by staff physicians to make sure that there are enough hospital patients to go around.

Creative diagnosis is a euphemism I coined to describe the indefensible behavior of doctors who keep themselves busy by finding disease where none exists. They do it by redefining the norms of health and sickness and employing other deceptions to create an artificial need for their services and those of their wondrous machines. Their eager allies in the medical-industrial complex are the drug companies, the equipment manufacturers, the testing laboratories, and even those friendly folks who manufacture infant formula and canned baby food.

I remember being amused years ago by pharmaceutical ads that defined constipation so broadly that unless you ate and slept in the bathroom you fell into the "irregular" class. The ads usually portrayed a middle-aged woman in a gingham housedress with a pained expression on her face. One hand was pressed against her hunched-over back, while the other pushed a vacuum cleaner or stirred a pot on the stove. Over the picture was a blazing caption, "CONSTIPATED?" that left no doubt about what the poor woman's problem was supposed to be.

I guess I was still too close to my own medical school brainwashing to be offended by the ad, but in retrospect I'm ashamed that I found it amusing. God knows how many millions of unconstipated women believed the ad's message about regularity and became instant candidates for the drug company's pills. Although the medicine itself was not particularly toxic, it was also worthless, and the means used to peddle it was a classic example of drug industry avarice and cynicism that has become commonplace today.

Almost no one seems to know it, because they've been educated by the ads, but there is no arbitrary standard for regularity. Unless you have physical symptoms of constipation, and you'll know if you do, it makes no difference whether you have a bowel movement three times a day or once a week. The damage is done when you are told you should have one daily, believe it, and take medications because you don't. You weren't constipated before you took the medicine, but once you're hooked on it you can be almost certain that it will so upset your normal rhythm that real constipation will result. That, of course, is precisely what the drug manufacturer wanted to achieve.

That's one example of *creative diagnosis*. Observe that the unsuspecting victims are persuaded that there's something wrong with them so they'll swallow a "cure" that will make them sick!

This is not an isolated example. Let me describe another variation of the same technique. One of the indications for the prescription of Valium—the most frequently used and abused drug in the country—is anxiety. Millions of normally anxious women are hooked on it by their doctors every year. It can be sold only by prescription, so while its sale enriches Roche Laboratories, it also enriches tens of thousands of doctors and pharmacists as well.

What does Valium do for the women who take it to relieve their anxiety? Well, the first of Valium's side effects is—guess what?—*anxiety!* The drug your doctor gives you to *relieve* anxiety also *produces* it, along with a generous helping of new symptoms as well. Take Valium to relieve anxiety and you may be rewarded with more anxiety, plus the potential side effects of confusion, constipation, depression, dizziness, drowsiness, fatigue, headache, incoordination, insomnia, jaundice, joint pain, libido changes, nausea, rage, rash, slurred speech, tremor, double vision, vision blurring, urinary incontinence, urine retention, and others.

The one that surprises me least is rage. Every woman who is put on Valium to relieve the normal stresses of everyday life should feel rage when she experiences some of the devastating side effects—or the addiction—that her doctor has wished on her.

Bendectin is another case in point. This toxic drug is prescribed for the relief of nausea and vomiting during pregnancy, although there is no solid scientific basis to believe that it works. Since nausea and vomiting are two of its side effects, it would be a miracle if it did work. But even more alarming is the fact that any doctor would ask a pregnant woman to risk diarrhea, dizziness, headache, irritability, rash, stomach pain, painful urination, vision blurring, and other more devastating side effects that I'll discuss later, in order to find out whether or not Bendectin works.

This sort of pharmaceutical creativity couldn't succeed and prosper, of course, if Modern Medicine decided to stamp it out. Prescription drug manufacturers couldn't sell their witches' brews if there weren't willing doctors to ladle them out. But don't expect the drug companies to go broke, because compared to doctors, the crime syndicate's pushers are pikers where drug abuse is concerned. Given the drug manufacturers' propensity to use the total populace as human guinea pigs, turning millions of circulatory systems into miniature Love Canals, doctors should be their leading adversaries. Obviously, they're not. Instead, Modern Medicine and the pharmaceutical industry are co-conspirators in advocating and dispensing the $19 billion worth of drugs—many of them dangerous, untested, and worthless—that are sold every year.

Meanwhile, in order to keep an oversupply of doctors busy, Modern Medicine has concocted no end of business development strategies of its own. Doctors have displayed incredible ingenuity in the use of creative diagnosis to manufacture nonexistent disorders simply by altering the previous norms. This strategy enables them to determine that normal physical characteristics are abnormal, minor ailments are major ones, inconsequential variations from questionable tests are indications of disaster, and small departures from standardized measurements are symptoms of life-threatening disease.

If you are like most Americans, you probably like to eat. It's a propensity we've developed because, unlike much of the world, there's a lot of rich food on our tables and most of it tastes pretty good. If you enjoy too much food too often, you inevitably become a little fat, and there's nothing really wrong with that. You may not even feel guilty about your weight if your husband diagnoses your condition as "pleasingly plump," hoping that you'll consider him "muscular," since he's no string bean, himself.

So you're both comfortable, well fed, and happy, right? Your life isn't upset by the agonies of rigorous self-denial, and the excess of adipose tissue is really nothing to worry about. Now, present your ample, healthy body to your doctor for a routine physical examination and see what happens: you're in trouble the minute you step on his scale! He peeks over your shoulder, compares your 150 pounds with the averages on his worthless chart, assumes a mournful expression, and shakes his head in dismay.

You walked into his office healthy, happy, and *pleasingly plump*. You leave it miserable, dejected, and *disgustingly obese*. You can consider yourself lucky if you don't also have a worthless and possibly dangerous prescription in your hand.

Without unduly laboring the point, let me suggest that almost endless opportunities for creative diagnosis are at your physician's disposal. Hypertension didn't attract much attention from doctors until the drug companies began making pills that gave Modern Medicine a profitable opportunity to intervene.

Hypertension is now interpreted by some screeners to include hordes of people who would have been considered healthy a few years ago. This justifies the administration of powerful, toxic medications with so many horrendous side effects that they make many of the dubiously hypertensive patients really sick. Many of them produce loss of libido and impotence and are, I suspect, responsible for more sexual dysfunction in the United States than psychological hang-ups.

If the blood pressure cuff doesn't give your doctor a reading high enough to declare that you're mildly hypertensive, he needn't despair. There's a good chance that your blood pressure will be low enough so that he can find you a victim of *hypotension,* a non-disease that was discredited nearly thirty years ago—long enough so that it can now be credibly revived. Forget that studies have shown that people with low blood pressure usually live longer. If your doctor *says* hypotension is a disease, it *is* a disease, and he'll probably treat it with shots of vitamin B-12. Even if hypotension *were* a disease, the shots wouldn't do any good.

You can also expect your doctor to cast a covetous eye on your kids. Educators who don't like unruly pupils have, with the willing help of doctors and psychologists, broadened the definition of hyperactivity to include a substantial percentage of those in the country who are under age twenty-one. As a consequence, for the comfort and convenience of teachers *and* parents, millions of normally lively kids have been drugged with Ritalin and turned into virtual zombies by its effects.

The time of life when doctors consider it safe to have children has been narrowed to the point where having babies is called unsafe at almost any age. Get pregnant when your doctor thinks you are too old or too young and he'll expose you to his whole bag of obstetrical tricks. Among them will be amniocentesis, a dangerous procedure that should be used sparingly, if at all, to determine abnormality of the fetus. Its staunchest advocates now recommend amniocentesis for all women over thirty. The indications for delivery by Caesarean section have been expanded so creatively that the section rate in some hospitals is now over 50 percent. Most of the indications are the result of analgesia, anesthesia, induced labor, and other intervention by the obstetrician in the natural process of birth.

All of this creative diagnosis is lucrative, of course. It keeps the drug factories humming and the hospital beds filled. It even makes the morticians break out in smiles. And it also makes doctors look good. The most striking example of this is the fact that a single pimple today is called acne, greatly enhancing the stature of dermatologists, who can now claim an 80 percent cure. That's almost as good as the concerned teenager could have obtained by staying away from the doctor and washing his or her face.

My friend John McKnight, a professor of urban studies at Northwestern University, looks at all of this with a probing and critical eye. He teaches that in the name of curing, caring, helping, and loving, increasing numbers of healthy people are being defined as sick. But behind this mask of service, he notes, lies the reality of servicers who need income—doctors, nurses, hospitals, drug manufacturers, pharmacists, and many others. Thus, "the client is less a person in need than a person who is needed," says John.

But what a price Americans pay to satisfy Modern Medicine's need!

A final warning: if your doctor is an expert at creative diagnosis, don't, for heaven's sake, ever tell him that you have a headache. Unless you have other symptoms that concern you, remind yourself that seven out of ten Americans take an analgesic to relieve a headache at least once a month. Keep your headache to yourself, because if you don't, you'll open a Pandora's Box of *possible* indications of serious disease. They'll be enough to keep your doctor, the laboratories, and maybe even the hospital, busy for weeks or months, subjecting you to a lengthy roster of expensive tests.

Your doctor knows that unless your headache is accompanied by a combination of additional symptoms it is probably psychogenic—a tension headache—and the best advice he can give you is to relax, take an aspirin, and go to bed. But if he's truly creative, and a mite unconscionable, your headache is the only excuse he needs to begin a search for an endless array of exciting diseases. They range from the innocuous common cold to cancer of the brain, but a host of others fall in between. Unless you crave attention, take a small gamble and assume that your headache isn't the result of chicken pox, diphtheria, scarlet fever, mumps, mononucleosis, influenza, pneumonia, hepatitis, sinusitis, tonsillitis, encephalitis, typhoid fever, brucellosis, dengue, Rocky Mountain spotted fever, leptospirosis, smallpox, yellow fever, tularemia, anthrax, malaria, meningitis, allergic rhinitis, gastroenteritis, polyps, hypoglycemia, hyperthyroidism, or cervical syndrome.

Headache is a symptom of all of these ailments, but chances are that you don't have any of them unless other symptoms are present—not even the one I forgot to mention, *the plague!*

3

"What Medical School Did *You* Go To?"

The less confidence your doctor has in the diagnosis he has made or the treatment he has recommended, the more likely he is to wave his sheepskin at you if you have the temerity to question his advice. "What medical school did *you* go to?" is the putdown he uses to dodge questions that he knows he can't answer to your satisfaction. Most of the time it works.

He doesn't use this ploy often. He doesn't have to, because most of his patients are too intimidated by his manner and his credentials to question the treatment he recommends. When he does use it, *beware,* because the odds are that he has given you some very bad advice.

Modern Medicine derives much of its power from the trusting and almost reverent attitude that most Americans have toward their doctors—toward *all* doctors. Roger G. Kennedy, director of the Smithsonian Museum of Technology, could have been talking about doctors when he said, "Positions of power are sheltered workshops for the ego." Power born of respect, much of it undeserved, is the rock on which the cathedral of Modern Medicine rests. The aura of omnipotence with which the medical establishment has surrounded itself deters you from inspecting your doctor closely enough to discover that he really has clay feet.

To escape the clutches of Modern Medicine, you'll have to deprogram yourself as you would if you were a captive of some dangerous cult. You'll have to get rid of the mental image you have of the kindly, competent, trustworthy, caring physician, and see your doctor as he really is. You'll find that he is not a real-life Robert Young, although he may be as good an actor, because medical schools do a better job training doctors to be actors than they do teaching them to keep you well.

During eight to ten years of medical education and training, doctors are taught how to make you believe they are God. After a few years of wielding enormous power over life and death, *they* begin to believe it, too. Most doctors would deny this, but once in a while one of them slips up and lets the cat out of the bag. In 1968, in his book strangely titled *The World of a Gynecologist,* Dr. Russell C. Scott had this to say about those who specialize in diseases peculiar to women:

> If, like all human beings, he is made in the image of the Almighty, and if he is kind, then his kindness and concern for his patient may provide her with *a glimpse of God.* (Italics added.)

A more searching look at your gynecologist might provide something other than "a glimpse of God." One of the surgical procedures most often performed without a clear indication of need is the hysterectomy. I'll have more to say about this procedure later, but it is worth noting here that the hysterectomy rate in England is only 40 percent that of the United States. That should tell you something about the creative diagnosis employed by American gynecologists.

In 1975, 1,700 of the 787,000 women who had hysterectomies in this country died as a result of the surgery. A *New York Times* analysis of data provided by the Commission on Hospital and Professional Activities, and by Dr. Eugene McCarthy of the Cornell University Medical College, revealed that surgery was not recommended by consultants in 22 percent of the cases they studied. Given the British experience, the probability is that the number that could have been avoided is far greater than that. But, simply accepting the 22-percent figure, it is apparent that 374 women died in 1975 as the result of hysterectomies that were not needed; on the basis of other studies, about 500 more died because of sloppy surgery and faulty techniques.

Some critics accuse gynecologists of performing "hip pocket hysterectomies" because the only real beneficiary is the surgeon's wallet. The wallets are fat, all right, but I'm convinced that most needless surgery is performed because of the passion for surgical intervention exhibited by those who teach in medical schools and because of the unswerving faith in the scalpel that is instilled in students during the surgical residency years. "When in doubt, take it out," is a common expression among surgeons. It has led me to counsel my students, tongue in cheek, that when they are confronted by an exam question on what treatment to use, they should always pick the most dangerous procedure in the book.

Jane Brody, medical writer for the *New York Times,* reported a case that demonstrates the hazards of gynecologists' devotion to surgical intervention, even when simpler, less costly, less dangerous, and equally effective alternatives are available. A young Florida woman who was troubled by backaches was advised to undergo surgery to have her "misplaced" uterus moved. The surgeon neglected to tell her how far he planned to move it, and when she emerged from the anesthetic she discovered that her uterus and one ovary had been removed. During the operation the surgeon damaged her bladder, so another operation was required to fix that.

I suppose that if the surgery had solved her problem she might have philosophically accepted her surgical nightmare as plain bad luck. However, when she had recovered from all the other pains the surgeon had inflicted on her, she still had the backache. In desperation, she finally visited an orthopedist, who examined her and found that one of her legs was shorter than the other. He put a lift in her shoe and the backache disappeared.

Do you suppose that the next time she saw her gynecologist she got "a glimpse of God"?

Every now and then the newspapers report the arrest of someone who has been practicing medicine without the formality of getting a license or even attending medical school. I can't recall a single instance in which the culprit was accused of injuring a patient, or in which he had not won the confidence and respect of the patients he treated. His offense lay in proving that you don't really have to go to medical school to be a successful doctor.

Even more dramatic examples of this principle are the cases in which surgeons themselves have sought assistance in the operating room from men who had never seen the inside of a medical school. Consider the case of Manuel A. Villafana, a poor boy from the South Bronx who became a multimillionaire by making and selling cardiac pacemakers and heart valves. In describing this high school graduate's astonishing success in the medical field, the *Wall Street Journal* noted that "the 39-year-old balding entrepreneur has earned a reputation in medical circles as a savvy salesman with a Midas touch." What an appropriate accolade for anyone associated with Modern Medicine, with or without an M.D.!

Mr. Villafana dropped out of Manhattan College at the end of one year and, after a succession of jobs, signed on as a salesman with Medtronic, Inc., a Minneapolis manufacturer of cardiac pacemakers. These devices are implanted surgically in the chest, where they supposedly keep the recipient's heart beating regularly by stimulating it with mild electric shocks.

"In 1969," according to the *Journal* article, "Medtronic sent Mr. Villafana to set up a South American sales office in Buenos Aires, and it was there that he began to develop a close rapport with doctors. Since pacemakers still were relatively new, Mr. Villafana says he frequently went into operating rooms and worked 'hand in hand' with doctors to implant the devices. 'They appreciated it,' he says. 'They didn't want to screw up.' "

What medical school did *he* go to?

In 1977, the district attorney of Suffolk County, New York, indicted two doctors, an anesthesiologist, a nurse, and a hospital for using unlicensed medical personnel to perform surgery. The prosecutor alleged that William McKay, a salesman of prosthetic devices who had only an eighth-grade education, was called off the golf course because of an emergency at the hospital. One of the devices he sold was being used there in a hip replacement operation being performed on Franklin Mirando. Here is McKay's account of the incident, which was reported in *Newsday*.

" 'I was on the golf course,' McKay said, 'when the assistant pro drove up in a golf cart and said there was an emergency. He drove me back to the pro shop and I called the hospital. I was told Mirando's hip had dislocated in the recovery room and the doctors were waiting for me before going back in. When I got to the OR [operating room], they told me to hurry up, scrub, and get into my greens.'

"McKay said that when he arrived in the operating room [the surgeon] told him to remove the artificial hip joint and put in another one. McKay said he spent 6½ hours redoing the surgery and tying together fragments of Mirando's femur."

Mirando, who filed a $2 million malpractice suit against the doctors because he wound up with one leg two inches shorter than the other, did not name McKay in his suit.

" 'Without him, I probably wouldn't be alive,' he said."

Where did Mr. McKay go to medical school?

The fact is that, when your doctor puts you down by boasting that he went to medical school, he really doesn't have much to boast about. I've been to medical school, and I've taught in several, and I'm trying to find a way to keep my grandchildren from finding that out. In all other areas of higher education the purpose is to expose the student to information and ideas that he can use to develop the capacity to think rationally, to reason, to question, to create. He is encouraged to debate with his professors and, when he applies for approval of his doctoral dissertation, he is expected to defend his thesis.

Not so in medical school. There students are taught to absorb doctrine without argument or question. They are taught to respond to their teachers in a reflex manner. For example, when he hears the word "streptococcus" the student is taught to respond with "penicillin." When the professor says "right lower quadrant pain" he is taught to respond "appendectomy," and God help him if he suggests that it might be a passing cramp. In short, medical school teaches the student a body of dogmatic material and restricts his right to exercise judgment to very narrow limits. He may be permitted to debate what kind of pertussis vaccine to use, but not to question whether whooping cough vaccine should be used at all. He may be allowed to disagree about the kind of antibiotic to use for ear infections, but not to question the use of antibiotics as standard treatment for infections, whatever their cause.

Virtually all of the major examinations in medical school are multiple-choice tests, so the student never has to write a single word, much less a sentence, a paragraph, or a page. That's why, when your doctor writes a prescription, you probably can't read what it says. Sometimes the pharmacist can't read it, either, and you're given a remedy for hypertension when your problem is gout.

I used to wonder why medical schools were so determined to make certain that their graduates couldn't write a legible word. After all, it would seem desirable for a doctor to write orders that a nurse can follow and prescriptions that a pharmacist can read. Now I think I have figured it out. If you examine the illegible scrawls in hospital records after the passage of time, it is almost impossible to identify the doctor who wrote an order or a report. That assures that the doctors who scribbled them won't suffer future liability for malpractice because of mistakes they made in the past.

The medical student who questions what is being taught will not be a favorite in the race to finish medical school, win a good internship and residency, and pass his license exams. Sometimes the hazards of rocking the boat can be even greater than that. I will never forget a student of mine who wanted to specialize in obstetrics but couldn't swallow all of the ridiculous obstetrical intervention that he was being taught. He began to ask questions of the obstetricians: Why were the mothers' feet up in stirrups? Why were they giving the women analgesia and anesthesia? Why were they inducing labor at such an early stage? Why were they performing Caesarean sections when there was no clear indication of need?

Did he get answers? No, but he got action. He was referred by the chairman of the department for a psychiatric examination, because any student who asks a hostile question in medical school is presumed to be "disturbed."

The tragedy of this dogmatic approach to medical education is not only that it screens out the most thoughtful, intelligent, and ethical students, or that it perpetuates traditional idiocies, but also that it virtually forestalls the application of creative noninterventionist approaches to medical practice. Dr. Roger J. Williams put it well in his book, *Nutrition Against Disease:*

> Medical schools in this country are now standardized (if not homogenized). A strong orthodoxy has developed that has without a doubt put a damper on the generation of challenging ideas. Since we all have one kind of medicine now—established medicine—all medical schools teach essentially the same things. The curricula are so full of supposedly necessary things that there is too little time or inclination to explore new approaches. It then becomes easy to drift into the convention that what is accepted is really and unalterably true. When science becomes orthodoxy, it ceases to be science. It ceases to search for the truth. It also becomes liable to error.

Remember that the next time your doctor asks you where you went to medical school. Ask him where *he* went to medical school, and then tell him you asked because you're going to see if you can find a doctor who went somewhere else.

4

"There, There, Dear, Don't Worry Your Pretty Little Head."

Ten years ago, while I was in charge of a teaching program in a major hospital, a woman medical student complained to me that she wasn't getting a fair shake from one of the attending physicians. She said he resented her because she was a woman and that he had actually told her that women shouldn't be taking up places in medical school. He maintained that sooner or later they would all go off to have babies and their education would go to waste.

I asked the student what she thought I should do about his sexist attitude, expecting her to suggest that I tell him to apologize to her and alter his behavior. Instead, she surprised me by insisting, with considerable fervor, that I fire him.

At first that seemed a bit harsh, but on reflection I decided that the request was reasonable, or at least not unreasonable. I told the offending doctor that he was going to be relieved of his service responsibilities. Well, *he* didn't think that was reasonable. He thought it so unreasonable that he complained to the head of the department, who didn't think it was reasonable, either.

He fired *me!*

His reaction probably shouldn't have surprised me, because the attitude displayed by both men permeates every aspect of Modern Medicine. And why not? There is no reason to expect doctors to be less chauvinistic than other men, and there are some powerful reasons why they are more so. Women *are* discriminated against in medical school, in hospitals, and in all other aspects of medical practice, and they are discriminated against and maltreated as patients. But they are also discriminated against in business, industry, government, education— even in religion. This attitude is wrong wherever you find it, but it is most unconscionable in medical practice. The chauvinism of a corporate manager may cost a woman a job, a raise, or a promotion, and probably some mental anguish over the manner in which she is treated in the workplace. *The chauvinism of a physician or surgeon, however, may condemn the same woman to a lifetime of dependence on drugs or cost her the life or health of her baby, to say nothing of the loss of her breasts, her uterus, her ovaries, and even her life.*

I can remember a time when nurses were taught to walk one step behind and one step to the left of the physician and to follow him in and out of elevators when he made his rounds. Today, nurses are harder to find than doctors, so most of that demeaning, overt sexism doesn't exist anymore. But the underlying attitude hasn't gone away; it has just gone underground. Doctors still view nurses as servants who are there to clean up after them, and they continue to resent women who strive for more exalted medical roles.

Women *are* accepted as professional technicians, but don't take that as evidence that the medical chauvinists are beginning to relent. On the contrary, the work women are allowed to do is dangerous work that men don't want and even studiously avoid. You've probably noticed that male doctors order x-rays and male radiologists read them, but they carefully maintain a safe distance from the radiology rooms. It is almost always a female technician who risks the radiation hazards that emanate from the infernal machines.

Another hazardous spot in every hospital is the operating room. Studies have shown that female anesthetists who are repeatedly exposed to the gases present during surgery are fifty times more likely than the average woman to develop breast cancer. They also have more miscarriages. And their children are sixty times as likely to develop cancer and four times as likely to be malformed at birth. The gases also impose some hazards on men. So who spends the most time inhaling them? Not the male surgeon and the male anesthesiologist, who arrive at the last minute and rush off as soon as the surgery has been done. The female nurses and anesthetists get there first, and at cleanup time, they are the ones who are left behind.

Women are granted the same kind of dubious opportunity in another high-risk area—the operation of artificial kidney machines. The incidence of hepatitis among the female technicians who perform renal dialysis is so high that some hospitals have removed the machines. But please note: where they are still in use, it isn't the male doctor who ordered the treatments who gets hepatitis; it is the female technician who handles the blood and operates the machines!

Little need be said about the historic discrimination against women who have sought admission to medical schools. Until recently, not even 10 percent of those entering United States medical schools each year were women. In 1979–80, almost 28 percent were female, but don't assume that this means Modern Medicine has had a change of heart. It is simply another case of avarice overcoming prejudice. Modern Medicine had a choice it could understand: admit more women or say good-bye to millions of dollars in federal aid!

Despite recent increases in female admissions, only one licensed physician in ten is a woman. Fewer than 5 percent of them were accepted for surgical residencies so that they could specialize in the area of medical practice that holds the greatest prestige and earns the greatest rewards. The median salary for the average woman physician is not quite $40,000 a year, compared to more than $67,000 annually for men.

The point I want to make about this discrimination is not so much that women are treated unfairly within the medical profession, although they certainly are. Rather, it is that sex discrimination practiced by male doctors toward the women in their ranks is also leveled against the women who entrust them with their care.

Some profound historic reasons have made sex discrimination more virulent in medicine than in any other professional field. As far back as Hippocrates' day, during the fifth and fourth centuries B.C., doctors believed that the female reproductive system was a source of hysteria and even insanity. For more than two thousand years, if a woman stepped out of the expected pattern of subservience and humility, her ovaries and uterus were blamed. The term *hysterectomy*, in fact, derives from the Greek word for hysteria (*hysterikos*), which means *suffering in the uterus*. Thus, to remove the uterus was to relieve the patient of hysteria.

In 1809 the first ovariectomy was performed, and throughout the nineteenth century gynecologists vied with each other to develop ever more radical forms of surgical invasion of the female anatomy. Having discovered the ovariectomy, the surgeons had to discover more reasons for performing it, so ovaries were routinely removed as a highly touted remedy for hysteria, psychological disorders, insanity, *and even to keep women under the social control of men*. These justifications for the performance of ovariectomies were used as recently as 1946!

Nineteenth-century medical literature is replete with references to the frailty and hysteria of women. If a woman rebelled against her husband's tyranny or failed to maintain an appropriately subservient and retiring family or social role, her reproductive organs were assumed to be the cause and castration the cure. In 1896 Dr. David Gilliam, one of many writers on the subject, praised the virtues of female castration as a means of securing obedience from women. He wrote:

Rohe, Morton, and others have blazed the way; and what do they tell us? They tell us that castration pays; that patients are improved, some of them cured; that the moral sense of the patient is elevated, that she becomes *tractable,* orderly, industrious, and cleanly. . . . My own experience in this line has been most happy. (Italics added.)

Ovariectomies are no longer performed for the ostensible purpose of making women more tractable and obedient, or at least it is unlikely that any gynecologist would admit that they are. But when you observe the number that are still performed without any evidence of medical need, you have to wonder whether some surgeons still enjoy doing them as a demonstration of masculine authority. Certainly Modern Medicine still views women as doctors always have: as weak, nervous, hysterical creatures, subject to all sorts of psychological ills related to the female anatomy.

That perspective dominates the medical treatment—or maltreatment—of women. It also produces a disparity in the treatment of the sexes that might have been modeled on the distinction made in Plato's Laws between the medical care provided slaves and that accorded freemen. The slave-doctor, according to Plato, prescribed "as if he had exact knowledge" and gave orders "like a tyrant." The doctor who catered to freemen went "into the nature of the disorder," entered "into discourse with the patients and his friends" and would not "prescribe for him until he has first convinced him."

Consider that dichotomy in light of the attitudes toward women displayed by two hospital residents quoted by Diane Scully in her powerful book *Men Who Control Women's Health.* One, an obstetrical/gynecological resident, said:

> I think we have less problems because our patients are women. I think women are easier to handle than men, easier to talk to, in a way. They listen more; they may even believe you. I think it is easier to treat them.

The other resident revealed the insensitivity that doctors display toward charity patients, especially women. These patients are too often viewed with animosity and scorn, treated as though they are subhuman, and denied any sense of caring or emotional support. This resident acknowledged that he felt that way, but said he knew he would have to change when he went into private practice and feared that might be hard to do. During my years of teaching I have known scores of interns and residents who felt exactly this way:

> You serve a different purpose in private practice. You are a father image or a psychiatrist or a friend, or something like that. Here we don't give that kind of service to patients. They don't expect it. A lot of what you do in private practice is that, plus figure out what you are going to do with your money, trying to make money. You are involved in different goals.
>
> Well, some people do it overnight. It's something that some people think is expected of them, and it can be a very phony, insincere thing. You know it's part of the image you might have to project. . . . People anticipate it and expect it. *So you smile and you call them dolly, sweety, pumpkin, things like that, and you pat them on the behind and you sort of talk down to them* and—uh—it's all very superficial. (Italics added.)

A nurse who read those quotations responded with a letter to *Mother Jones* magazine, citing a few quotations from her own experience in the obstetrical/gynecological sections of a large university hospital. She said that, while comments of this sort weren't made by all male physicians, they usually thought they were funny when they were made by others. Her examples:

A resident anesthesiologist: "I can't stand it when these Lamaze mothers come in for delivery. If they don't want anesthesia when I'm ready for it, it screws up my timing. They will want it later, though, but that's the time I make sure I get there *damn* slow—on *my* time."

From a resident in obstetrics and gynecology: "For Halloween I'm going to cover myself with slime and go as a woman."

An attending physician, after examining an adolescent patient: "Well, this confirms my theory about adolescent pregnancy. They all have big boobs."

Some students of medical history, among them G. J. Barker Benfield, who wrote *The Horrors of the Half-Known Life,* argue that the gynecological specialty was developed as a means of retaliation against and control of women. Doctors, he asserts, resented the entry of women into the work force during the Industrial Revolution and the women's rights movements that were associated with this new freedom. They exploited their power as physicians to retaliate against and control women who were challenging male dominance. They did it by performing aggressive surgery, such as clitoridectomies and ovariectomies, as a means of showing women who was boss.

The aggressive surgical intervention that was developed in early gynecology was the forerunner of widespread and often needless surgery that is found in all fields of surgery today. But where needless surgery is concerned—perhaps because they've been at it longer—gynecologists and obstetricians are still the worst of the lot.

I have always found it fascinating and appropriate that one of those early gynecologists, Dr. J. Marion Sims, is revered by contemporary practitioners as "the father of gynecology." The basis for this recognition was Sims' role as founder of the New York Women's Hospital, as inventor of a number of surgical instruments, and, most significant, as developer of a surgical technique to close vesicovaginal fistulas, a condition in which there is an opening between the bladder and the vagina. The latter achievement also won him another title—"The Architect of the Vagina."

When Sims died, the *Journal of the American Medical Association* was extravagant in its praise: "His memory the whole profession loves to honor, for by his genius and devotion to medical science he advanced it in its resources to relieve human suffering as much, if not more, than any man who has lived within this century."

Who was this compassionate genius? Sims became a general practitioner in the South in 1835. Initially, he shared with other physicians of the time a distaste for gynecological problems and avoided treating them. He was led into the field by chance, when he became intrigued with the case of a female slave named Anarcha, who developed a vesicovaginal fistula because of instrument damage Sims inflicted on her while delivering a baby.

Remember that this was an era during which female slaves were valued mainly for the babies they could produce, an era when some plantations were huge slave-breeding farms. Sims knew that because Anarcha was no longer able to bear children, her value had been destroyed by the damage he had done. He also knew that countless other black females were considered "worthless" because of the same condition.

Sims decided to begin a program of research to discover a surgical remedy for vesicovaginal fistula, utilizing female slaves as his research subjects. He built a small hospital/laboratory and had no trouble securing Anarcha and six other similarly afflicted female subjects from their cooperative owners. Between 1845 and 1849, he experimented on these unfortunate black women, trying various procedures to close their fistulas.

Sims operated repeatedly on his slave-subjects, *working without anesthetic* but keeping them heavily dosed with opium, which probably explains why they didn't run away. He finally perfected his technique during an operation on Anarcha, who had inspired his work in the first place. This was the great humanitarian achievement for which Sims is still honored today. Long forgotten is Anarcha, the poor woman on whom Sims operated, without anesthetic, *thirty times!*

Anyone who closely observes the reckless intervention that prevails in obstetrical-gynecological practice will conclude that Sims is an appropriate choice for recognition as "the father of gynecology." His obsession with surgery and his lack of compassion for the women who endured the incredible torture he inflicted on them are still reflected in the behavior of many who practice this specialty today.

Sims' use of women as human guinea pigs was not unique to his time. Modern Medicine and its pharmaceutical allies are still experimenting on unsuspecting victims who number in the millions. Many of them are damaged by the drugs they are given and some of them die.

A critic of this wholesale human experimentation, Dr. Herbert Ratner, the former director of public health in Oak Park, Illinois, once observed with delicious sarcasm that women are the best guinea pigs Modern Medicine can find. He says they take the Pill without asking any questions, pay for the privilege of taking it, and are the only experimental animals known who feed themselves and keep their own cages clean.

Women are so cooperative, of course, because they assume that doctors are cautious, conscientious, caring professionals whom they can trust. How well-placed is this confidence? Consider the following examples:

Between January 1971, when it was introduced, and June 1974, when it was removed from the market at the request of the Food and Drug Administration, an intrauterine device (IUD) called the Dalkon Shield was installed by doctors in about 4 million women—2½ million of them in the United States. It was done despite the fact that the IUD had been tested inadequately, and it almost immediately began producing dangerous side effects in the women who wore it.

It is now estimated that 1,100,000 women in the United States have suffered an acute pelvic infection due to an IUD since 1970. One in five of them is sterile as a result, and at least seventeen women have died as a consequence of wearing the device. It was not until September 1980, after its insurance companies had paid out $55 million to the Dalkon Shield's victims—with more than 600 court actions and more than 300 claims still pending—that the manufacturer, A. H. Robins Company, wrote to physicians urging them to remove the shields from the patients who were still wearing them. After all the publicity about the shield's hazards, there's a message in the fact that such a letter to physicians was considered necessary so late in the game.

Between 1940 and the early 1970s the synthetic female hormone diethylstilbestrol (DES) was widely prescribed to prevent miscarriage. No one really knew whether it would prevent miscarriage, or what the long-term side effects might be, because the drug hadn't been tested enough to find out. But that didn't dissuade the drug company from marketing this unproven drug or prevent doctors from prescribing it for millions of women.

Eventually a study was conducted at the University of Chicago Medical Center to determine the effectiveness of DES. More than 2,000 healthy, young, pregnant women were given the drug but led to believe that it was a vitamin supplement. They were not told the name of the drug or that they were human guinea pigs participating in an experiment. The study confirmed what was already suspected—that DES was ineffective in preventing miscarriage. However, even that evidence failed to halt its manufacture or persuade doctors that it should no longer be prescribed.

By 1972 the long-term side effects of DES began to appear. It produced cancer of the breast in some of the women who took it and caused vaginal cancer in some of their female children and genital abnormalities in some of the male children to whom they gave birth.

To their credit, those who conducted the experiment tracked down as many of the women as they could find who had unwittingly participated and warned them of their plight. Meanwhile, the children of those mothers who received DES from their obstetricians are also at risk, yet Modern Medicine has been unwilling to devise a system to track them down and warn them of the hazard they face.

Every young woman whose mother took DES should be warned that she will increase the risk of vaginal cancer if she takes female hormones like Premarin or birth control pills. Every doctor who prescribed DES has a moral obligation to search his files to identify the patients who received it and alert them and their children that they are at risk. However, given the costs of doing so, and the potential of such warnings as a source of malpractice suits, it is unlikely that many doctors will part with their money to save their victims' lives.

It is no coincidence that some of the worst examples of callous experimentation on unsuspecting women involve new forms of birth control. A few years ago a subcommittee of the United States Senate investigated reports of damaging and even deadly side effects from the Pill. Dr. Philip Ball, an Indiana internist, testified that Modern Medicine, in prescribing the birth control pill for more than a decade, had been conducting "a massive, double blind, uncontrolled experiment," with 50 million women as human guinea pigs.

Dr. Hugh J. Davis, assistant professor of obstetrics and gynecology at Johns Hopkins University School of Medicine, deplored the fact that women who took birth control pills were not adequately warned of the risks. "In many clinics," he said, "the Pill has been served up as if it were no more hazardous than chewing gum."

You may ask why doctors would subject their female patients to these risks. It seems illogical, given the fact that the prevention of birth deprives the obstetricians of a lot of revenue. Dr. Ball answered the question when he told the senators, "The sacred birth control pill has had the halo of being the drug that would control the massive social problems of a burgeoning population. It could be used on the poor, ignorant, illiterate women who scarcely knew what birth control was all about."

Dr. Ratner expressed the same view regarding the Pill when he testified that it was foisted on American women "because it was promoted as the solution to the population problem in the undeveloped countries and to the growing welfare problem in the U.S."

This squares with my own conviction about Modern Medicine's penchant for social engineering at the expense of the traditional medical ethic, "First, do no harm." It is clear to me that present-day physicians will do almost anything to prevent women from having babies, particularly if they are black or brown, uneducated, or poor. They have been so brainwashed by the population-control zealots that no price—even experimentation on millions of women—is too high to pay to lower the birth rate among welfare mothers or in the underdeveloped countries of the world. Thus they abandon their medical oath and rationalize involuntary sterilization in charity hospitals, needless hysterectomies, cancer-causing hormones, unsafe and untested IUDs, and every other means of birth control that they or the drug manufacturers can invent.

Any woman who is even mildly attracted to this concept of

indiscriminate population control should ask herself whether she wants her doctor to play God. Should Modern Medicine sponsor a two-pronged attack on the population explosion by killing some women in order to prevent the birth of others? Before answering that question, every woman should ask herself whether she would accept the proposition if her own life were one of those at stake. It is, because Modern Medicine has demonstrated time and again that the experiments it begins on the poor ultimately are inflicted on all, even the rich.

Some of Modern Medicine's most exotic surgical abominations, in fact, appear to have been invented *only* for the rich, or at least for those affluent enough to stay off the welfare rolls. One is the pet procedure of a gynecologist in Dayton, Ohio, that fortunately is not widely shared.

Apparently, the doctor is convinced that when God designed the female genitalia He made a terrible mistake. He put the clitoris in the wrong place. But not to worry: for $1,500 the surgeon and his trusty scalpel will give God a belated hand. He'll embellish your sex life and help you achieve maximum orgasmic potential by creating what some critics have called the Mark II vagina. You can then look forward to the ultimate in sexual fulfillment because your clitoris will be located where the doctor thinks it belongs.

According to the doctor, more than 4,000 women have had this surgery, including some patients on whom he performed the operation without bothering to ask whether or not they wanted it.

Another specialty that concentrates primarily on women, and is replete with abuse, is plastic surgery. I see women in the course of my own medical practice who are troubled by their marital relationships and desperate to know what has gone wrong. Some attribute their problems to the fact that their physical attributes no longer qualify them as models for the cover of *Vogue*.

Now and then these troubled women seek my advice on whether a visit to a plastic surgeon might revitalize a dying marriage and make them attractive to their husbands again. I can assure you that I don't encourage them. Other than that performed to correct real, traumatizing disfigurement, I think much plastic surgery is the biggest rip-off on the medical scene.

I'm not alone in that view. It is shared, among others, by Dr. Elizabeth Morgan, who is a plastic surgeon herself. In her book, *The Making of a Woman Surgeon,* Dr. Morgan deplores the fact that some members of her specialty behave as though they were hairdressers and "give the field a bad name."

Dr. Morgan cites the case of one board-certified plastic surgeon who passes out his business card in supermarkets, and another who told a female guest at a party that he could make her eyes more beautiful.

"Still another," she writes, "told a woman, who just wanted a couple of moles removed from her face, that he could give her a package deal for $3,500 and fix up her nose and baggy eyes. I saw the woman, and there was nothing wrong with her nose and her eyes."

The inexcusable tragedy lies in the large proportion of costly plastic surgery that is performed on women who hold the expectation that it will not only change their features, but also salvage their messed-up lives. The psychological impact of their subsequent disillusionment—something the surgeon could have anticipated if he had explored the patient's motivation for plastic surgery rather than grasping for a fancy fee—is almost certain to produce a state of mental depression even deeper than the one they suffered before.

In a discussion of sexism in medicine, one of my friends expressed the belief—based on her own experience—that, while doctors are instinctively chauvinistic, they do mirror the attitudes of the patient and respond to their perception of the behavior and expectations of the patient. It is imperative, therefore, that you make it clear at the outset that maintaining your health is a partnership agreement with your doctor in which you hold the controlling vote.

Don't reinforce your doctor's feelings of omnipotence by allowing or encouraging him to patronize and intimidate you. Be on your guard, and make him explain and defend every diagnosis he makes, every drug he prescribes, every operation he recommends. Don't be in awe of him. Compel him to accept you as an equal, because you deserve his respect at least as much as he merits yours!

5

"I'm Going to Order
a Few Simple Tests."

Every woman is familiar with loss leaders—the items that merchants advertise below cost so that they can lure you into the store to sell you something else. For decades the loss leader of Modern Medicine has been the annual physical exam. It is the device doctors employ to get their hands on perfectly healthy people so that they can declare that they are sick.

There's no doubt that this strategy has been a conspicuous success. Unless you are remarkably resistant to high-pressure salesmanship, you probably share the belief of most Americans that an annual physical examination is necessary to protect your health. Modern Medicine has used all of its resources to sell this concept, aided by organizations like the American Cancer Society and its ubiquitous slogan, "Fight cancer with a checkup and a check."

Not until 1980 did the American Medical Association and the American Cancer Society finally acknowledge what I have been chastised for saying for years: *annual physical examinations, when they are performed on symptomless patients, probably do more harm than good.*

Don't expect either organization to publicize greatly this change of heart. However, in 1980 the AMA did finally abandon its support for the routine annual physical and the American Cancer Society for routine annual mammography, Pap smears, and chest x-rays. It took too long, but they had to cave in because of the overwhelming evidence that these procedures are actually dangerous, not just no good.

Many studies done over the last decade or so have established that the annual physical examination is a waste of money and a waste of time. One of the most extensive was conducted between 1964 and 1973 by the Kaiser Health Plan in California. They identified members of their health plan who were between the ages of thirty-five and fifty-four and from comparable economic and social backgrounds. Half of them were urged to come in regularly for physical examinations, and the others were not. After seven years of observation, the study determined that the overall health of the two groups remained the same—in terms of both mortality and disease—whether or not they had a periodic physical examination.

My concern about these examinations, and the tests that are routinely associated with them, is not simply that they are largely worthless. I'm concerned because too often they lead to physical damage and even death.

The Pap test is a classic example of this. Although it had never been subjected to adequate study to determine its effectiveness, this test for cervical cancer was eagerly accepted by Modern Medicine. A 1973 study found that more than half of all American women over age seventeen had taken the test during the previous year.

Gynecologists welcomed the Pap test because it gave them access to their patients at least once a year. Although numerous studies questioned its value, doctors had no incentive to discourage annual testing, because it provided them with so many opportunities to intervene. If they were questioned about the value of the test, they simply pointed to the declining death rates from cancer of the cervix as evidence of the value of the Pap smear.

In rationalizing the routine annual use of the test, they ignored a ten-year-old reference that questioned its worth. In this report, Drs. C. L. Sharp and Harry Keen pointed out:

> Several studies have shown declining death rates from cancer of the cervix, but since these were evident even before cytologic detection (Pap smear) was commonly in use, there is as yet no conclusive evidence that this type of detection method has played a definite part in reducing mortality.

Recently, two female researchers, Dr. Anne-Marie Foltz of New York University and Jennifer L. Kelsey, Ph.D., an epidemiologist at the Yale University School of Medicine, also reported that there was no conclusive evidence that the annual screening of millions of women had reduced the death rate from cervical cancer. They pointed out that the test was notoriously inaccurate, and had never been subjected to controlled trials to determine its effectiveness.

My concern is not so much directed at the efficacy of the Pap test in preventing cancer deaths as it is with the number of deaths and the amount of damage it has *caused*. A few years ago I was approached by a friend—a well-known physician himself—whose wife had undergone a Pap smear. Cancer was suspected, and she was being urged to have a conization. This is the biopsy procedure that is routinely performed after a questionable Pap test, and he asked me whether I thought she should have it done.

I told him I didn't see any point in it. They had been married for thirty-five years, she had never been on the Pill or taken any postmenopausal estrogens, and there were no other reasons why she should be at risk. Consequently, it seemed pointless to proceed.

Not surprisingly, because most doctors believe the myths that Modern Medicine creates, he advised his wife to go ahead with the biopsy procedure. As I had expected, the results were negative, but she bled so much that she had to have an emergency hysterectomy. During the hysterectomy she went into shock, which required the transfusion of several pints of blood. This led, six weeks later, to serum hepatitis from which she almost died.

What a price to pay for submitting to an unnecessary, inaccurate, routine test!

At about the same time, the wives of two other friends of mine had routine mammography exams. One of them had positive indications of a tumor, so a biopsy was done. A positive reading from the biopsy came back from the lab, and the woman's breast was removed. The postoperative pathology report showed no evidence of cancer of the breast. The other patient also showed evidence of a tumor, but the biopsy was negative. She breathed a sigh of relief and nothing further was done. The biopsy report proved to be erroneous, and she *died* of cancer of the breast.

I realize that these are isolated examples from which no scientific conclusions can be drawn. I cite them merely to dramatize the reasons routine examination and testing of apparently healthy people is so hazardous to their health. It is because they lead to radical medical or surgical intervention based on tests that are suspect at best and grossly inaccurate at worst. They also lead to sloppy medical practice in which inadequate tests are substituted for careful clinical evaluation and sound medical judgment.

As in the case of the Pap smear, many of the tests that doctors routinely administer are inaccurate and unproven to begin with, and these deficiencies are compounded by false interpretation and inefficient, careless work in the labs. The Pap tests produce false negative results about 20 percent of the time, giving doctors and women who actually have cervical cancer confidence that they don't. On the other side of the coin, false positive results occur in 5 to 10 percent of the tests that are given. This accounts, in part, for the nation's soaring hysterectomy rate.

Even when the tests themselves are valid, the odds are great

.аt the lab to which they are sent will mess up the results. Medical testing laboratories are scandalously inaccurate. In 1975, the federal Center for Disease Control (CDC) surveyed labs across the country and found that 10 to 40 percent of their work in bacteriologic testing was unsatisfactory, 12 to 18 percent erred in blood grouping and typing, and 20 to 30 percent botched hemoglobin and serum electrolyte tests. Overall, erroneous results were obtained in more than a quarter of all the tests. The consequence was the administration or withholding of medical treatment and lost income that resulted in a great deal of needless human suffering and cost the nation's economy $25 billion a year.

In another nationwide survey, 50 percent of the high standard labs licensed for Medicare work failed to pass. A large-scale retesting of 25,000 analyses made by 225 New Jersey labs revealed that only 20 percent of them produced acceptable results more than 90 percent of the time. Only half passed the test 75 percent of the time. In the labs studied by the CDC, 10 to 12 percent of the healthy specimens were reported to be diseased, causing patients to receive hazardous treatments when they were not really sick!

Many of the expensive tests that are administered in the course of a routine physical examination have little, if any, value, even when the labs come up with the correct result. A 1975 study was made of the value of twenty different blood tests routinely given to patients on admission to hospitals. Of the one thousand cases investigated, the tests were of benefit to only one patient. The Canadian Task Force on the Periodic Health Examination, which has recommended against annual physical examinations, also concluded that routine electrocardiograms, blood chemistry tests, and even urinalysis tests were not worthwhile. The hazard of all routine testing, of course, is that while an occasional patient may benefit, many more may suffer because their tests yielded inaccurate results.

Even the routine measurements that are taken in the course of a physical examination—weight and temperature, for example—can hurt the patient more than they help. If you are running a fever, the doctor prescribes aspirin to bring it down.

This defies the basic physiological principle that I learned in second-year high school biology, but that they apparently still haven't caught up with in medical school, which is that fever promotes phagocytic activity by the white cells so they can gulp up the bacteria that are making you ill. It makes no sense to interfere with this process by reducing body temperature, unless it reaches the danger zone. I rarely prescribe aspirin to reduce temperature except in extreme cases, and they have to be plenty extreme.

It makes no sense to become upset about a symptom that simply means the body is hard at work fighting off disease. High body temperatures are actually induced artificially in the treatment of cancer and other forms of disease. Yet when a mother calls about a sick child, the first thing most doctors ask is whether she has taken the child's temperature and how high the reading was. The doctor can't learn much that is useful from that question because many innocuous diseases—roseola, for example—produce very high temperatures but are nothing to worry about. Other life-threatening diseases, such as tuberculous meningitis, are often not accompanied by any fever at all.

Although knowing a child's temperature is of little value from a medical standpoint, it may have one value for you. If you are having trouble getting an appointment with your pediatrician, remind yourself that he's been programmed to believe that temperatures are important, even though he doesn't know why. If you want to be sure that he'll see you promptly, and he asks about your child's temperature, tell him that it's 106. That may raise some questions when you reach the doctor's office, but a few white lies will handle them, and your doctor can get at the business of finding out why your child is sick.

One of the most common reasons for taking children to pediatricians is the simple sore throat. You've probably been taught by Modern Medicine that sore throats may mean streptococcic infection and, in turn, the rheumatic fever to which it is supposed to lead.

As far as I'm concerned, this whole strep routine is nothing more than a mirage—one that produces what I used to call the *hundred-dollar disease*. I felt that way a few years ago, so by now it is probably a $200 disease. Why is it a mirage? I'll give you two reasons. First, there is no sound scientific evidence that strep leads to rheumatic fever, a disease that rarely appears except among the very poor. Second, most mothers don't know, but doctors should, that during the winter months 20 percent of all children carry strep bacilli in their throats—without any symptoms—at one time or another. However, this does not mean that they have the disease.

A competent physician can tell clinically whether or not a patient has a *real* strep infection. There are three cardinal signs: high fever, pus in the back of the throat, and large, swollen neck glands.

But what actually happens when you take your child to the pediatrician because he or she has a sore throat? The doctor promptly converts the extreme into the mean and orders a throat culture, regardless of the clinical signs. In one out of five cases the test will reveal the presence of strep bacilli, and the doctor will make the illogical leap to the conclusion that the positive test means that the sore throat is due to strep. In the doctor's mind, strep means a prescription for penicillin, which the child must take faithfully for ten days or it will do no good. The doctor may also order a urinalysis to make sure the child doesn't have nephritis, and he will certainly order you to come back at the end of ten days for another throat culture to determine whether the penicillin has done its work.

If you are like four out of five mothers whose children are given penicillin, or who are told to take it themselves, the chances are that the medicine won't be administered faithfully for the full ten days. In that case, although it may help avoid early complications such as sinus infection, it does not prevent the possibility of more serious later complications such as rheumatic fever and nephritis. But the sore throat clears up anyway, leaving you out the price of the penicillin, two throat cultures, and two office visits, but grateful to the doctor who "cured" a non-disease.

This misuse of testing procedures is costly to the patient but relatively harmless in terms of the patient's health. There are many situations, though, in which the routine substitution of tests for clinical evaluation and judgment presents real hazards for the patient the doctor is supposed to help. This might not be the case if all tests were valid scientifically and interpreted accurately, but too often they are not. When a doctor neglects clinical evaluation and relies too heavily on tests, you are at risk because of the potential inaccuracy of the tests. On one hand, you may have a disease that is left untreated. On the other, you may be the victim of treatment or surgery that you didn't need.

When testing becomes a matter of routine, the doctor is apt to stop thinking because he depends on the test. The stage beyond that is the one in which he stops looking at the results, as though his work were done when he ordered the test. Do you find that incredible? Then explain an experiment in which a laboratory returned to doctors hundreds of reports on serology tests that showed positive indications of syphilis. In only three or four cases did the doctors follow up and order a recheck on the results of the tests! Obviously, the others had not read the reports or they would have done so, to fulfill their medical responsibility to their patients, and their legal obligation to health authorities to report the results of the tests.

In my experience there is almost an inverse relationship between the clinical skills of a doctor and the extent to which he relies on tests. Many doctors today take a cursory history from their patient, give an even more cursory physical examination, and then order a whole battery of tests.

This is tragic because it means that the most reliable means of diagnosis are being ignored. My experience, and that of every doctor I respect, is that about 75 percent of patients can be diagnosed on the basis of the history alone, another 15 percent from the physical examination, and 5 percent from the laboratory tests. The remaining patients have ailments that don't get diagnosed by any of these methods.

Obviously, given these percentages, doctors should place

their greatest trust in the traditional means of diagnosis. Why don't they? I think the reasons are fairly obvious, although I can't read the minds of my peers. Taking really complete histories and giving really thorough physical examinations are the most time-consuming and least income-producing diagnostic procedures that a doctor can employ.

Doctors who want to maximize their profits can save their own time and vastly increase their profits by installing a lot of fancy diagnostic equipment and hiring underpaid women to perform batteries of tests. For example, some practices are now equipped with electroencephalograph (EEG) machines. Although studies have shown that an EEG will neither diagnose nor rule out epilepsy, and that it is not helpful in the diagnosis of minimal brain damage, doctors who own the equipment keep it busy doing tests of this kind. A 1977 study by two Johns Hopkins neurologist-pediatricians said that EEGs are "currently much abused and much overutilized," and added, "The profitability of the tests has led to a proliferation of machines in neurologists' offices and a consequent increase in the number of tests run by uncertified electroencephalographers."

Little wonder that the practitioners of Modern Medicine ordered 8 billion tests in 1975, which alone produced an income of 15 billion dollars that year!

6

"Let's Just Take a Couple of Pictures."

One of the most dangerous weapons in Modern Medicine's arsenal is the x-ray machine. Most doctors order x-rays carelessly and needlessly and either don't know or don't care about their damaging cumulative effects. You should fear a doctor with an x-ray machine as you would a six-year-old waving a loaded gun.

All Americans are threatened by the indiscriminate use of x-ray machines, but more often than not they are pointed at women. *Women are twice as likely as men to get cancer from their potentially deadly radiation effects.*

Most doctors won't warn you that x-rays can produce cancer in your breasts or leukemia in your unborn child. If you ask them about the hazards, they'll give you the same assurances that I was given more than thirty years ago by my professors in medical school. They'll tell you that the radiation is at such a low level that it can't do any harm.

That's just as much hogwash today as it was then. Any doctor should know that there is no minimum level of radiation

49

below which a woman is safe from harm. He also should know that the radiation effects are cumulative, so it isn't just the dose you get from a single x-ray that's important—you can be damaged or destroyed by the combined effects of all the x-ray doses you have ever received.

How sinister that is! You go through life with your doctor and your dentist piling the effects of one x-ray on top of the others. You don't know they are irrevocably harming you until twenty or thirty years later, when the breast cancer caused by the accumulated low-level radiation appears.

Doctors are fond of telling you the obvious, that x-rays are valuable to diagnose or treat life-threatening disease. But, as Dr. Karl Z. Morgan, head of the Oak Ridge National Laboratory health physics department has said, they are "one of the most misused of medical tools." Your doctor won't tell you how misused they are, but you are entitled to know, so I will.

Item: Thirty percent of the x-rays taken in the United States—*nearly 300 million a year*—are ordered in cases where there is no valid medical need.

Item: Another federal expert says that if carelessly done and unnecessary x-rays were reduced by one-third, it would save the lives of 1,000 people who die of cancer every year.

Item: The genetic effects of one year of x-ray radiation may lead to as many as 30,000 deaths in future years.

Why are all Americans, and women in particular, exposed to so many needless x-rays? There are many reasons, none of which make doctors look very good. Some are given as a part of the ritual of Modern Medicine. The physician demonstrates that he can look inside your body so that you will regard him with awe. A whole series of x-rays is often taken as part of survey examinations, "just in case" they may turn up something that the doctor missed in his clinical examination. Some are given needlessly as a routine part of hospital admission, or because of bureaucratic government requirements for certain types of jobs. Large numbers are given by employers, as an irrational part of routine annual executive physicals or preemployment exams.

Doctors also order x-rays—at your expense—as a defense against potential malpractice suits, even when there is no medical need. Many are ordered, along with countless other tests, because they enable the doctor to make three times as much money while doing less work. Doctors who refer their patients to radiologists order only half as many x-rays as those who profit from owning their own x-ray machines.

Don't forget that an x-ray is an x-ray, whether it is a doctor or a dentist who owns the machine. Over the years I have heard from scores of women who were concerned about the possible effects of dental x-rays on women of childbearing age. When one woman, whose dentist took x-rays routinely on each of her visits every six months, finally expressed concern about being exposed to radiation so often, the dentist laughed at her fears, insisting that the radiation dosage was so minimal that even the cumulative effects couldn't do any harm.

That dentist's attitude is common throughout the profession, and it defies the policy of the American Dental Association (ADA), to which most dentists belong. Acknowledging that the cumulative effects of x-rays are dangerous, the ADA cautions dentists against the routine use of diagnostic x-rays, warning that they should only be used "after careful consideration of both the dental and the general health needs of the patient."

Despite that admonition, I have yet to find a woman whose dentist has expressed any interest in her medical history or in how much other radiation she has had. I haven't even found one whose dentist bothered to determine whether she—knowingly or not—was pregnant before his assistant turned on the machine.

To make matters worse, not one dentist in a thousand knows the dosage to which his patients are being exposed, and, in fact, studies have shown that a third of all dentists expose their patients to twice as high a radiation dose as is necessary. That's true of x-ray operations in large hospitals, as well.

It is bad enough that the average American woman is exposed to six times as much radiation as the typical British citizen, and at least twice as much as the average Japanese or

Swede. The hazards of this senseless radiation exposure are multiplied because in over 90 percent of these x-ray examinations, the patient is provided with no protective shielding at all.

The risks are also increased because most x-ray equipment is not inspected regularly, because an incredible proportion of the units are defective, and because some are not inspected at all. Fire extinguishers are more closely inspected than x-ray machines. Studies have shown that a very high proportion of x-ray units deliver excessive amounts of radiation, and that many expose women to extra radiation dosage because of too large a beam. Women are too often subjected to dental x-rays that radiate their breasts as well as their jaw.

In many states x-ray equipment can be operated by anyone who walks off the street. Only one state—California—requires all persons who give x-rays, whether technicians or doctors, to pass a state examination. Only a few even bother to license x-ray technicians. The result is that many x-rays are given by receptionists, bookkeepers, and other office personnel who are untrained in keeping x-ray exposures at the minimum level. They may deliver a radiation dose that is 100 times the amount required, increasing the threat of cancer or genetic damage.

What it all boils down to is simply this: Every year, in the United States, millions of women are exposed to cancer because their doctors order unnecessary x-rays given by incompetent operators using defective machines!

That's not all the bad news. The horrendous risks don't even end there. Modern Medicine's track record is little if any better in the interpretation of x-ray films. Once the x-ray has been taken, there is a ridiculously high probability that an incorrect diagnosis will result. Thirty years ago studies showed that about 25 percent of radiologists differed with each other in the interpretation of the same chest film. When they were tricked into rereading the same film, *31 percent of them disagreed with themselves.* Studies in 1955, 1959, and 1979 produced similar results. The accuracy rate of radiologists hadn't improved significantly in all those years!

This shocking degree of error in interpretation can result in terribly adverse consequences for the women whose films are misdiagnosed. If disease is found where none exists, the patient may be subjected to dangerous surgery or other treatment she doesn't need. Many women who have lost their breasts because of tumors that proved to be benign can testify to that.

The risks are also high if you look at the other side of the coin. If no disease is found where it does exist, the patient and the doctor may be lulled into a false sense of security. The patient is not treated for a disease that could have been detected if the doctor had used other diagnostic means. Women die every day for both of these reasons, as well as from the risks imposed by the x-rays themselves.

Pregnant women need to be particularly cautious where x-rays are concerned. It is known that a single abdominal x-ray of a pregnant woman can predispose her child to leukemia. And remember, the danger is there whether the abdominal x-ray was ordered by a doctor, or whether you get one accidentally from an incompetent operator who doesn't know which way to point the machine.

The initial finding of a relationship between leukemia and prenatal x-rays goes back to the 1950s, yet one 1966 study revealed that 26 percent of all pregnant women were exposed to medical x-rays. More unconscionable is the fact that there are still obstetricians who take unnecessary pelvimetric x-rays to determine the size of the pelvis, and others who don't trust their own skill at palpation of the abdomen and order x-rays to determine the position of the fetus. The poor baby is subjected to radiation before it is even born!

Irresponsible medical practice of this sort is so ludicrous it can only stem from ignorance or stupidity. Whenever I hear of one of these cases I am reminded of the old story about the butcher who sold brains. He got a dollar a pound for pediatricians' brains, but for obstetricians' brains he charged five dollars a pound. When a customer asked him why obstetricians' brains were worth so much more, he explained: "Do you know how many obstetricians' brains it takes to make a pound?" (Pediatricians aren't much smarter, and they are certainly no more ethical. Despite their benign and concerned manner, you won't find them telling a mother that her obstetrician injured her child. I remember being taught in medical school never to look back at what caused a deformed child. That was the obstetrician's business and I shouldn't interfere. The reason is obvious. Pediatricians depend on referrals from obstetricians, and they don't dare lay blame on the obstetricians because they'd be out of business if they did.)

Women of childbearing age have a special need to be concerned about the cumulative effects of the x-rays they receive during the course of their lives. Doctors don't like to admit it, because it is Modern Medicine's fault, but it is accumulated radiation, not age in and of itself, that influences the birth of a child with Down's syndrome.

Many doctors continue to preach the conventional belief that older women who become pregnant are at increased risk, because of "tired eggs," that their baby will be a victim of Down's syndrome. Nonsense! There may be tired husbands and tired wives, but I don't believe there are "tired eggs" any more than I believe there are "tired sperm."

If a woman has accumulated much radiation during her life, there is an increased risk that she will deliver a baby with Down's syndrome. Yet, despite overwhelming evidence that this is the case, doctors continue to tell all older women that they shouldn't have babies because their eggs may be weary, rather than determining how much radiation exposure they have had.

I keep hoping that the mounting evidence that x-rays kill and damage people will lead doctors to curtail their use. However, I know that these hopes are nothing more than wishful thinking on my part. If anything, the trend is going in the opposite direction, as x-ray equipment proliferates, and as the equipment manufacturers develop ever more powerful and dangerous x-ray machines.

It is a sordid indictment of Modern Medicine, but Americans will continue to be exposed to excessive x-rays because the economic incentives to keep the machines busy are far too great. The best I can hope for is that doctors will exercise greater discretion in the use of x-rays on pregnant women. The *Journal* of the American Medical Association in May, 1974, pointing out "the potential ability of ionizing radiation to cause congenital abnormalities," urged them to do just that. It even laid down these rules:

1. Assume a woman in the reproductive years is pregnant unless proved otherwise.

2. If a woman may be in the first trimester of pregnancy, avoid inclusion of the pelvis in the primary x-ray beam if at all possible.

3. Where feasible, always shield the pelvis and abdomen of women when performing diagnostic roentgenographic studies.

4. If there is valid medical indication to perform a diagnostic study using radiation on a pregnant woman, this will generally outweigh the remote possibility of harm to the patient or her fetus.

5. If a woman receives a relatively high amount of radiation (5 to 15 rads) to the pelvis in the first trimester of pregnancy, the increased risk of a congenital anomaly is from 1 percent to 3 percent. Such a risk may justify a therapeutic abortion. On the other hand, if the parents are psychologically able to handle the slight increased risk of a malformed child, one can recommend that the pregnancy continue.

The AMA recommendations are a step in the right direction, but given the breadth and magnitude of the total x-ray threat, they don't go nearly far enough. Doctors should use x-rays as sparingly as possible, and certainly *never* in cases where an adequate diagnosis can be established clinically. They should warn women about the potential cumulative effects of radiation. They should help their patients to determine the extent of previous radiation exposure and to establish a running record of how much radiation they have received.

Doctors are always trying to convince their patients to change the dangerous behavior—smoking, for example—that the *patients* control. Isn't it about time doctors begin to do something about the dangerous behavior that *they* control?

In the absence of any inclination on the part of Modern Medicine to curtail the use of x-rays, what can you do to defend yourself? First, bear in mind that most doctors are so accustomed to ordering x-rays on the slightest provocation that they do it without even stopping to think. Your best line of defense is to force the doctor to question whether the x-ray he is ordering is one he really needs. You can do that by asking some questions of him. Try these:

1. What are you looking for?
2. What are the chances that you'll find it if you take these x-rays?
3. Can you find what you are looking for by some less hazardous means?
4. If you find it, is it something you can treat?
5. Does the treatment entail any risks? If not, why can't you just assume I have the condition, skip the x-ray, give me that treatment, and see if it works?
6. When was the last time your x-ray equipment was checked for safety?
7. Will it be operated by a trained technician who knows what he or she is doing and will keep the radiation dosage to a minimum?
8. What form of shielding or other protection will you furnish me?
9. What dose of radiation will I receive?

If your doctor is honest and conscientious, and not a medical prima donna, he'll answer these questions in a way that will enable you to decide whether or not you want to have the x-rays. In the course of answering them, *he* may even have second thoughts. But if he is evasive or antagonistic because you have dared to question his judgment, watch out. He may be ordering a procedure that you don't need.

That's when you can take advantage of the fact that you're a woman. You don't have to tell him you don't trust him. Just tell him you don't want an x-ray because you think you are pregnant. Unless he's a complete idiot, that should be that!

7

"Take These and You'll Feel Better."

The creative diagnosis employed by doctors and the creative marketing that fills hospital beds do untold damage to your health and your pocketbook. However, they can't hold a Bunsen burner to the creativity of the American drug manufacturers. Every year their research laboratories pour out a toxic stream of new chemicals and compounds which they market as "ethical drugs" by creating unethical non-diseases that they can be used to treat. Most of these useless and dangerous prescriptions are written for women.

Your morning newspaper often features headlines lauding a new "miracle drug" that has just appeared. You may find this reassuring, but you shouldn't. Most of these heralded discoveries are miracle drugs, all right, but not in the sense the manufacturers would have you believe. The miracle is that our overmedicated society has survived all of the so-called miracles the drug companies and doctors have shoved down our throats. A more objective look at the toxic miracles that doctors boast about reveals a sinister fact: An inordinate number of this year's drugs were developed to cure the damage caused by a miracle drug that was proudly announced in some previous year. Repeatedly, new drugs are sold to counter the symptoms produced by others. And so the miracles continue, eternally enriching physicians, surgeons, druggists, and the pharmaceutical companies, at a horrible cost in dollars and lives.

An incredible example is the major tranquilizer, Thorazine, which is prescribed for psychotic disorders, nausea and vomiting, tetanus, agitation, excessive anxiety, and tension. One of its side effects is extrapyramidal reactions—symptoms resembling those of Parkinson's disease. When this side effect appears, it is treated with Artane, which has the side effects of dizziness, nausea, psychotic manifestations, delusions and hallucinations, mental confusion, agitation, and disturbed behavior.

The indicated treatment for a woman who suffers from Artane's side effects is—what else?—Thorazine! The drug is like a kitten chasing its own tail, only it isn't a kitten, or even a cat. It's a tiger, and a dangerous one at that. You may—and should—wonder how a woman's health can be improved by a drug that produces the very symptoms it is supposed to cure.

An incredible percentage of the medicines doctors prescribe—possibly three out of five—simply don't work. Many are prescribed for purposes for which they were not intended. Far too many are prescribed in place of safer and more effective alternatives, and most of them are given to women.

Hundreds of drugs are being marketed without conclusive evidence that they will do no harm, and others would not even be on the market if the manufacturers had not concealed evidence that they *will* do harm. Drugs that are relatively safe in some applications cause fetal abnormalities or mental retardation when they are prescribed—as they too often are—for pregnant women. An unknown number hold a long-term potential for inducing cancer of the breast, cervix, or other organs that may not become apparent until years later when those who have used them begin dying from their effects.

Most drugs reach the market after being subjected to animal tests, and the first human testing they get is when your doctor tests them on you. There is inherent danger in every one of these drugs, yet only about one in twenty is a significant improvement over the drug it is intended to replace. Most drugs are not developed to enrich your life, but to enrich those who make, prescribe, and sell them.

You would not be threatened by dangerous prescription drugs, of course, were it not for the laziness, carelessness, greed, or ignorance of the doctors who prescribe them. No woman should accept a prescription from her doctor without questioning its worth. Remind yourself that medicine hasn't changed since two centuries ago when Voltaire wrote, "Physicians have been pouring drugs about which they know little for diseases about which they know less into human beings about whom they know nothing." That warning is even more appropriate today because there are so many more drugs to abuse.

Not only do physicians prescribe drugs with great abandon, but they rarely give their patients much, if any, information about dangerous potential side effects—such as sudden death— that are often worse than the disease the drug is supposed to cure. If they did, many production lines in the drug factories would come to a screeching halt.

A physician in one of my television audiences rationalized this failure to communicate the bad news about drugs with this defense: "I agree that patients should be given some information about side effects, but you can't give them so much that you scare them to death." In other words, it is all right to tell a woman that a drug might make her nauseous, but, for heaven's sake, don't tell her that it might also cause convulsions, heart failure, or anaphylactic shock! Tens of thousands of patients die every year from the side effects of drugs. I'm confounded by the perverse logic that doctors shouldn't tell their patients the drugs they are being given might kill them, because the information might *scare* them to death. When women are given the opportunity to make an informed choice, what they *do* know won't kill them, but too often what they *don't* know will!

The chauvinistic belief of most doctors that women are weak, hysterical creatures, given to perpetual anxiety and depression, is mirrored in the abuses that female patients suffer. Many doctors relate to women as though they functioned on the same intellectual plane as their kids. The kids fare better than the women, though, because at the end of the office visit they get a free lollipop. Their mothers are handed prescriptions for expensive and risky happiness pills.

I don't know how many kids are hooked on lollipops, but I do know how many American women have been hooked by their doctors on psycho-active drugs. In 1978, a federal official told a congressional committee that 36 million women were taking tranquilizers, 16 million were on sedatives, and 12 million were being drugged by stimulants—mostly worthless diet pills. During 1978, 12 million new women victims were lured onto this medical merry-go-round when their doctors gave them their first prescriptions for mood-altering drugs.

Doctors wrote 160 million prescriptions for tranquilizers, sedatives, and stimulants in 1979. Only about 10 percent of them were written by psychiatrists, the only medical specialists who are trained to recognize their effects. A federal report found that 60 percent of the mind-altering drugs, 71 percent of the antidepressants, and 80 percent of the amphetamines are prescribed for women. Women are prescribed more than twice the quantity of drugs as men for the same psychological symptoms.

The same study revealed that in 1976 doctors wrote 27 million prescriptions for sleeping pills—*a billion doses* all told. They were responsible for about 25,000 harrowing trips to hospital emergency rooms, and 5,000 of the victims failed to leave the hospital alive. Dr. Robert Du Pont, director of the National Institute on Drug Abuse, was shocked by the number and appalled by the realization that 5,000 unfortunate souls were dead because they took pills that "are probably not effective in terms of treating insomnia." Studies by the National Academy of Sciences and other reputable scientific groups agree that sleeping pills are both dangerous and ineffective, except, of course, when they put you to sleep so effectively that you never wake up!

Congresswoman Cardiss Collins of Illinois, head of a congressional task force on women and drugs, is one of many public officials concerned about the tendency of doctors to lure unsuspecting women into dependence on tranquilizers and other prescription drugs. She says:

> We are all prone to thinking of drug abuse in terms of the male population and illicit drugs such as heroin, cocaine, and marijuana. It may surprise you to learn that a greater problem exists with some 2 million women dependent on legal prescription drugs.
>
> It is not uncommon for a doctor to advise a male patient to "work out" his problems in the gym or on the golf course, while a female with the same symptoms is likely to be given a prescription for Valium.

Congresswoman Collins no doubt singled out Valium for the obvious reason that it is the most used—and abused—drug in the country. My friend John McKnight says that the major transaction in Modern Medicine is a male doctor giving a female patient a mood-modifying drug. Valium alone produces about half a billion dollars a year in sales for Roche Laboratories and about *50,000 patients a year for hospital emergency rooms.* Along with other tranquilizers, sometimes combined with alcohol, it was responsible for 1,500 emergency room deaths in 1978. There's no available body count on its victims who died at home or in the street.

As a group, tranquilizers are the cause of twice as many hospital emergency room visits by overdosed users as are heroin and cocaine. Ninety percent of the patients seen on these visits are women. Says FDA Commissioner Jere E. Goyan:

> I think we need to cut back on these uses of tranquilizers that merely deal with anxiety. These drugs were never intended for that purpose. I'm especially concerned about people who have

become addicted to these drugs without even knowing that they are. Women, particularly, seem to be the victims.

We're talking about some 5 billion tranquilizer pills that are prescribed every year. (Italics added.)

Tranquilizers, as Dr. Goyan notes, were not originally intended to treat simple anxiety. They were developed for use in mental hospitals to reduce or replace the electroconvulsive shock treatments and brain surgery being used on severely psychotic patients.

It's a long leap from a violent patient in a locked ward of a mental hospital to the sunny kitchen of a mildly anxious suburban housewife. But doctors made the transition, validating my most important premise—in Modern Medicine anything that can be done will be done to any available victim. The drug companies, of course, eagerly pushed the doctors along this disastrous path, lighting a beacon every step of the way.

The doctor's brainwashing about drugs begins in medical school, where the modest amount of information he gets from professors is overshadowed by the aggressive "education" he gets from drug company detail men. These pharmaceutical predators blanket the campus with literature promoting the products their companies sell, provide the students with free medical kits, textbooks, supplies for their parties, and even research grants and summer jobs.

This medical school indoctrination accustoms the doctor to accepting a similar relationship in private practice after he finishes medical school. Detail men call regularly on physicians, providing gifts and samples and hyping them about the alleged virtues of the drugs they sell. It has been estimated that the amount spent by drug manufacturers to promote their nostrums to the medical profession amounts to about $5,000 per doctor per year. Drug companies spend an estimated $1.3 billion annually—13 percent of their total sales revenues—promoting their products. The average doctor gets a shower of gifts—desk sets, briefcases, paperweights, calendars, etc.—from pharmaceutical companies. They also gave away *3 billion pills,* 8,500 for each physician in the land. In contrast, only 9 percent of sales revenues was spent on research, most of it aimed at finding new pills to peddle, not to determine whether the ones they already sell are dangerous or really work. Millions of dollars are also spent on surveys to determine the effectiveness of pharmaceutical promotion and to devise marketing strategies that will help the manufacturers shove additional billions of pills down American throats.

An ally of the detail men is the pharmacist, who also has an enormous stake in their efforts to urge doctors to prescribe the maximum number of pills. Consequently, many pharmacists conspire to inform the detail men about which of their powerful poisons are most popular with each of the doctors in the area that they serve. This enables the drug salesmen to concentrate their efforts on the doctors who have been least receptive to the potions they sell.

The performance of the detail men is closely monitored to be certain that they are faithfully applying their employers' devious marketing techniques. *Unbelievably, the monitors are not drug company supervisors. They're the customers, the doctors themselves.* Many doctors have been enlisted in a cadre of so-called reporting physicians, who surreptitiously fill out reports on the performance of the salesmen who visit them. Their reward is the prestige they gain when the drug manufacturer contributes $10 per report to their medical schools in their names.

As a young medical student, and even as a young doctor, I naively believed that the army of detail men who were on the road representing drug manufacturers were there to help me save lives. It didn't take me long to realize that this wasn't the primary motive of pharmaceutical manufacturers. They're out to make money and to make everyone *think* their products will save lives.

Month after month I watched detail men march into my office, armed with samples and elaborately expensive literature describing new products in glowing, exaggerated, and sometimes deceptive terms. Of course, they knew and I knew that many of these drugs were dangerous, untested on humans, and possibly ineffective for the purposes for which they were to be prescribed. As I got to know them better, many of them confessed that what they were doing made them sick.

When doctors aren't being brainwashed by detail men, they are besieged with the same sales pitch when they read the medical journal ads. If you pick up a copy of the *Journal of the American Medical Association,* you'll find it littered, from cover to cover, with three-, four-, and five-page tranquilizer ads. Printed in eye-catching full color, they are usually profusely illustrated, and the message they convey is printed in very large type—except for the warnings about side effects, which they don't want the doctors to read. The models in the photos are miserable-looking females who might have been recruited from among the surviving models for the 1930 issue of *Vogue.*

In 1978, a representative of the Pharmaceutical Manufacturers Association was asked about the unappealing, dejected models used in these tranquilizer ads. He replied that "Illustrations in medical ads, as in all ads, are designed to attract the attention of the reader. They typically will depict individuals whom the physician will relate to in his own practice—people like those he's seen in his own office."

Muriel Nellis, author of *The Female Fix,* recalls hearing the head of a major medical advertising firm tell how his company, through artful language and marketing campaigns, has helped "enlarge the whole concept of illness" in order to create a market for mood-altering drugs. He seemed blissfully unaware of what a damning indictment of the drug industry this admission was.

The technique by which this has been accomplished is revealed in the captions that accompany the depressing models in the tranquilizer ads. They feature as symptoms of non-diseases almost every transitory mood and emotion known to women. The use of tranquilizers is advocated to help mothers cope with the problems of raising children, and with the empty nest syndrome when the same children leave home. They are also touted for relief of the tensions of marital problems, financial difficulties, a move to a new town, a new job, a new assignment in a job, midlife crisis, social demands, "measuring up," the pressures of institutional life, or apprehension about virtually all of the problems that trouble any normal woman.

In their search for a broader market, the pharmaceutical companies are even willing to encourage doctors to inflict tranquilizers on kids. In an ad for Vistaril, Pfizer suggested its use to deal with childhood anxieties. Staring out of the ad is a little girl with tears streaming down her face. The caption reads: "School, the Dark, Separation, Dental Visits, Monsters."

I don't know what monsters Pfizer was talking about, but knowing that one of the many side effects of Vistaril is convulsions, I don't need to tell you who I think the monsters are!

The ritual belief that every office visit must end with a prescription also affects the behavior of doctors. When presented with a patient who has psychological problems that they don't want to or can't treat, they give the patient a tranquilizer whether or not its use is indicated. Studies of Valium and Librium use have shown that three-fourths of the prescriptions written were for conditions inconsistent with the approved use of these drugs. Dr. Donald Rucker, professor in the Ohio State University School of Pharmacy, says he is "unaware of a single study in the literature able to document that prescriptions of psychoactive agents corresponded with standards of rational use established by the investigators." Doctors prescribe these drugs freely but know so little about them that in one study of Librium, half of the doctors asked to identify its active ingredients couldn't do so.

The extent to which drug company promotion has influenced medical beliefs and behavior and caused physicians to think of tranquilizers as cure-alls, was brought home to me quite forcefully when I picked up my daily newspaper one day last year. In it was a column, written by a fellow medical columnist, that began with this letter:

Dear Doctor: In the last year, I have had swellings in different parts of my body, especially the face and lips. I was in the hospital for a week, where the swelling was diagnosed as an allergy.

I have to eliminate certain foods (chocolate, nuts, eggs, fish, citrus fruits) from my meals.

The day after I was released from the hospital, the swelling appeared again. I don't know what I'm fighting. Can you give me any advice?

Mr. A. J.

The doctor-columnist's reply:

Rather than eliminate all those foods at once, it might be best to do it systematically, one at a time. In this way, you may be able to track down the specific offender.

You also may have to check out other notorious allergy-producing foods like wheat and milk. And you can't overlook drugs.

Sound advice, if he had stopped there, but he didn't. His reply continued:

Allergies are pretty tricky things. Nerves can be a factor. It's not uncommon for nervousness to tip the scales and allow an allergy to a specific food to pop up.

You probably are a breadwinner, who began worrying about how all this would affect your work when you came home from the hospital. *Perhaps a mild tranquilizer will help you.* (Italics added.)

Note that the man who wrote the letter had not complained about a psychological problem. The columnist creatively diagnosed that problem by mail, without seeing or talking to him. The columnist warned, rightly, against the possibility of an allergy to drugs. Then, having read the mind of a correspondent whom he had never examined, after guessing at his occupation, and without exploring the drug allergies he had alluded to, the columnist prescribed a tranquilizer to cure a non-disease in a patient he had never met.

No wonder tranquilizers are selling at the rate of a billion dollars a year!

For many doctors and many patients, Valium has become the

real-life equivalent of the "soma" described by Aldous Huxley in *Brave New World.* You may recall that it was "the perfect drug . . . euphoric, narcotic, pleasantly hallucinant," possessing "all the advantages of Christianity and alcohol and none of their defects." Valium does, indeed, have most of these qualities, but don't for a moment believe that it is without defects.

"There's a need for Valium, but not for a mass of people to take it," according to Dr. Darryl Inama, director of the pharmaceutical service at the Haight-Asbury Free Clinic in San Francisco. He goes on:

> It causes subtle, unseen habituation. People go to see doctors for family problems or for self-identity, and instead of sending them to counseling, overworked physicians find it much easier to tell them, "I'll give you a pill and you'll feel better," rather than facing the problem directly and trying to deal with it.

Although Roche Laboratories, the manufacturer of Valium and Librium, has denied that either drug is addictive, the *Physician's Desk Reference,* which is compiled from information supplied by manufacturers, warns that persons taking "excessive doses" of Valium over a long period of time may experience withdrawal symptoms if they abruptly discontinue taking the drug. These symptoms may include "convulsions, tremor, abdominal and muscle cramps, vomiting, and sweating."

What are you, if not addicted, when in order to get off a drug you have to go through that?

No one can tell Dr. Barry Rumack, at the Rocky Mountain Poison Center in Denver, that tranquilizers aren't addictive. He treats fifty persons a month for tranquilizer addictions and gets monthly inquiries from up to 500 others. He says:

> It is a crutch. When we had the old doc running around on horseback he could talk to his patients. Now we tend to give drugs. If you see a doctor now for nerves, he gives you something rather than talk to you for thirty minutes.

If you take 80 to 120 milligrams of Valium a day for forty to sixty days, you are hooked. Most doctors don't prescribe that much, but people go to several doctors, figuring if some makes them feel good, more will make them feel better.

Doctors like it because it keeps patients quiet and happy. Patients like it because it makes them feel good.

He might have added, "The manufacturer likes it because it is making his company rich."

Some of the most heart-rending letters I receive from readers of my monthly newsletter are from women whose doctors have hooked them on tranquilizers or other drugs. Many of them are scared to death because of what the drugs have done to them, but can't stand the withdrawal effects when they try to give them up. What would you tell the victim in this tragic case?

In 1958 I developed hypoglycemia and, since I was holding down a heavy job and was having trouble sleeping, my doctor prescribed a 10-mg. Librium tablet at bedtime. That helped for a while but later lost its effect. Other medications were prescribed, but I couldn't tolerate any of them—they made me groggy all the next day. So I finally settled for waking up at 3 A.M. and staying awake the rest of the night.

When this doctor died, I turned to another one who, after hearing about my sleeping difficulties, suggested that 200 mg. of Placidyl might be effective. I tried it, and he was right. I have been taking both Librium and Placidyl ever since.

Recently, I developed arthritis in my knee, and the doctor prescribed Motrin. It was invaluable in the beginning, but after a while I started to develop side effects. The doctor suggested I take Ascriptin, which seems to control the arthritis very well. When I stopped taking Motrin, my doctor suggested I also stop taking Librium. That happened about a month ago, and afterwards I developed a swimming sensation in my head as well as heaviness in both my head and chest. I also started to feel very shaky, so he put me back on Librium, and my condition improved.

Could I have become addicted to Librium and Placidyl? I found it impossible to sleep after I stopped the Librium. What do you think about my predicament?

I told the lady I at one time used the word "incredible" when I heard of extremely bad cases, but no longer did so because I had heard so many bad cases I now use "incredible" only when I hear something good. Beyond that there was little I could tell her except that withdrawal symptoms after prolonged use of Librium and Placidyl are well-documented, and both products are clearly labeled as having the potential for developing psychological and physiological dependence.

A junkie is a junkie, whether she is using legal or illegal drugs. Her only course was to find a doctor who would help her through the withdrawal process so she could get off the drugs.

A 22-year-old woman wrote that she had been on tranquilizers since having a nervous breakdown several years before.

I've been on Elavil, Haldol, Norpramin, Sinequan, and Triavil. I stopped taking all of them last October, and I went through withdrawal—nausea, stomach cramps, diarrhea. *When I complained of these symptoms my doctor wanted me to take still stronger drugs.*

I'm going to be married soon. What should I do? I don't want to start this vicious circle all over again. (Italics added.)

Her doctor had turned her into a walking pharmacy, and there was nothing I could tell this poor woman other than that there was no easy way out. I wrote:

Other than the fact that your drug supply was doctor-prescribed, your situation hardly differs from that of the ordinary street addict.

Your sensible attitude has already successfully led you through the cold-turkey treatment, and you are responsibly trying to reject resuming the habit. Your next step is to rid yourself of the drug pusher, even if he happens to be your friendly physician.

I'm still shocked when I receive letters like this, although I get hundreds of them every year. But shock turns to fury when I hear from pregnant women whose doctors are giving them tranquilizers and other dangerous drugs. They not only damage the mothers but also risk inflicting deformities on the unborn child. I find this outrageously callous and stupid in the face of strong evidence of a link between tranquilizer use and birth defects.

In 1976, the FDA ordered pharmaceutical companies to advise doctors to avoid prescribing four major tranquilizers to pregnant women, citing this possible link with birth defects when these drugs are taken in early pregnancy. Obviously, the manufacturers weren't happy about it, because Valium, Librium, Miltown, and Equanil represent about $1 billion in annual sales to their manufacturers and are the most widely used drugs in the world.

Years earlier, between 1959 and 1965, a facility of the Kaiser-Permanente medical program reported 1,096 births to women medically diagnosed as anxious, tense, or mildly depressed. A study of these cases revealed that 402 of these women had been given the tranquilizer meprobamate, which is sold under the trade names of Miltown and Equanil. Another 175 received chlordiazepoxide (Librium). The study found that seventeen of the Miltown/Equanil users and nine of the Librium users had babies with severe birth defects. This was a combined rate of about 12 per 100, compared to a rate of 4.6 among children whose mothers took other drugs and 2.6 among those whose mothers took no drugs at all.

Although the drug manufacturers objected to the study as not significant, Dr. Carl Leventhal, deputy director of the FDA Bureau of Drugs, said, "Unless a drug has been specifically demonstrated as safe in pregnancy, it should be used only with caution. Any drug should be used only where there is clear medical benefit. The vast majority of drugs have not been specifically studied, and physicians should be very cautious in prescribing them."

There are few situations in which the administration of a drug during pregnancy can be justified. It may be necessary if it is essential to the mother's health or to treat an illness that threatens the child. Unfortunately, Modern Medicine does not limit the prescription of drugs to these situations. Most doctors—ill-trained in pharmacology except by drug company salesmen, whose educational efforts can scarcely be considered objective—prescribe drugs for pregnant women far too freely. It is currently estimated that the typical pregnant woman receives an average of four drugs during her pregnancy, most of which entail a known or unknown potential risk to the fetus.

Recently, one of my readers wrote expressing concern about the possible effects on her baby of the *six* drugs she was given during her pregnancy to treat the symptoms of a persistent cough and cold. The prescribing information for one of the drugs warns specifically against its use during pregnancy because it can pass from the mother into the unborn child. Doctors are warned against the use of one of the others because its safety during pregnancy has not been established. Had any of the drugs been used to deal with a life-threatening situation, their use might have been justified, but that was not the case. The most any of them could do was to make her cold symptoms a bit more bearable, which certainly could not be construed as a reason for risking the health of her unborn child.

Drugs can harm the fetus at any stage in its development, but the danger of physical anomalies or mental damage is greatest during the first trimester of pregnancy. This is the period when the development of the major organs occurs. The central nervous system, brain, and spinal cord are formed during the period between 2 and 5½ weeks after conception. The heart, kidneys, and blood vessels develop during the period between 2½ and 6 weeks after conception. The arms and legs develop between the third and eighth weeks, the liver and intestines between the third and fourteenth weeks, the palate between the fifth and twelfth weeks, the eyes and ears after the first 3½ weeks. The time of greatest risk for other parts of the body, including the face and lungs, is still unknown.

Obstetricians are more inclined to seek the approval of the mother by displaying concern for her comfort than to protect the welfare of her unborn child. It is vital, therefore, that pregnant women educate themselves about drugs and try to avoid taking them throughout their pregnancy, because even after the first trimester there is still a great unknown risk. The obstetrician should not give the mother's comfort precedence over the life and health of her unborn baby. Admittedly, this may make life more difficult for the mother, who may legitimately long for a magic pill to alleviate one or another of the discomforts that accompany pregnancy, but few informed mothers will risk their child's future for that reason. Danger lurks in every medication, whether intended for coughs and colds, constipation, relief of pain, insomnia, stomach distress, or symptoms of anxiety or depression.

Evidence that aspirin can dramatically arrest the growth of human embryo cells was demonstrated a decade ago in a study done in England. The effects of aspirin include fetal deaths, birth defects, and bleeding in the newborn. Female sex hormones, including the Pill, if taken during pregnancy, have been shown to double the rate of congenital heart defects. High doses of vitamin C can produce jaundice, and high doses of vitamin K can cause mental retardation. An anticoagulant named Coumadin has been shown to increase the risk of miscarriage. Dilantin, prescribed to treat epilepsy, can result in abnormal metabolism of folic acid, a vitamin needed for normal development of the fetus. Reserpine, given for hypertension, may interfere with the baby's ability to control body temperature and withstand stress. In some cases, diuretics have been found to reduce the baby's oxygen supply and affect its brain.

Antacids that contain bromides and sodium may provide so much salt to the baby that they lead to fluid retention in the fetus. Mineral oil, taken as a laxative, may reduce the absorption of vitamin K by the fetus and cause bleeding in the newborn. The hazards of cold and cough medicines have not been proven, which is reason enough not to take them since they provide nothing but temporary relief of symptoms and do nothing to cure a cold.

Finally, the use of tranquilizers during pregnancy—or at any other time, for that matter—should be avoided as the plague that they are. Although specific effects have not been fully documented, the hazards of mood-modifying drugs are sufficient to cause the FDA to issue the warning that "while these data do not provide conclusive evidence that minor tranquilizers cause fetal abnormalities, they do suggest such an association. . . ."

You owe it to your baby not to expose the fetus to that risk!

If all of the drugs marketed by the pharmaceutical manufacturers were useful, effective, and safe, their marketing practices would still be reprehensible, but many drugs are not. Moreover, the federal Food and Drug Administration, which is charged with keeping unsafe drugs off the market, is so handcuffed by the political influence of the drug companies that the protection it affords is more illusory than real. Its powers are too weak, its consultant experts are too often captives of the drug industry, and its payroll is loaded with ex-employees of the pharmaceutical companies who still have their ex-employers' interests at heart.

Prior to the introduction of a new drug, the FDA has the power to require evidence, from animal tests, that it appears to be safe. The FDA can also require that the manufacturer prove that the drug lives up to the claims that are made of it. Note that this does not require the company to prove that the drug provides significant benefits that outweigh its risks. It must merely do what they say it will do.

On the basis of animal experimentation, the drug is ultimately introduced to the market with the approval of the FDA. The animal experiments are paid for by the companies that are regulated. In order to get approval, they occasionally have falsified the results. FDA approval is the starting gun for a massive program of involuntary human testing to determine whether, when given to humans, the drug does not harm them and also works. The manufacturer and its willing allies, the doctors, race full speed ahead to sell as much of the drug as possible to their human guinea pigs before evidence begins to appear that it is killing or injuring some of them or that it doesn't work.

Often, after a new drug is introduced, independent scientific researchers begin conducting additional animal tests. Frequently, they discover what the manufacturer's research didn't find—or found but concealed: the drug produces cancer in laboratory animals. Almost invariably the manufacturer, who persuaded the FDA to approve his noxious product on the basis of animal tests, has a convenient change of heart. He resists removal of the drug from the market by arguing that the evidence that it is killing his customers is inconclusive because it was based on animal tests.

What an incredible double standard! Drugs are routinely approved for use by humans on the basis of inconclusive animal tests, but the manufacturers then insist that they shouldn't be removed from the market unless there is conclusive evidence based on human victims that they are unsafe.

The concept of retaining innocence until guilt is proven is quite appropriate in the field of jurisprudence, because it may save innocent lives. However, it is totally inappropriate in pharmacology where every day it is *sacrificing* innocent lives. But the laws are such that questionable, worthless, or dangerous drugs can stay on the market for decades while the industry successfully resists all efforts of the FDA to have them removed. Meanwhile, those who take them are suffering physical damage that may not become visible for years.

We will not know for another twenty years whether the chemicals introduced in the 1960s were hazardous [says Dr. Irving J. Selikoff, director of the environmental sciences laboratory at Mount Sinai Hospital in New York]. We need better methods than we now have to identify things without waiting to see the dead bodies in the street. . . . At the moment we're very insecure about some of our animal studies, because what happens in a rat is not necessarily what happens in a mouse. But it's not all that bad. Because if it causes cancer in mice, and then successively in rats, hamsters, guinea pigs, and dogs, one would have to be very brave to say it's not going to happen in man.

What we do not want to do is pay for new products at the expense of human illness and human disease and human life. We have no evidence at this time that any exposure to a cancer-producing agent is absolutely safe.

The political influence wielded by the pharmaceutical industry is awesome. It has persuaded Congress to maintain such limited authority to regulate the industry that it virtually checkmates the FDA. The Environmental Protection Agency has been granted the power to protect people from chemical pollution of the natural environment by other major industries. Yet, Congress won't give the FDA the authority it needs to prevent the doctors and the drug companies from pouring dangerous, inadequately tested chemicals directly into the bloodstreams of the same human beings.

Medical history is replete with examples of the impotence of the FDA. The most recent example came in September 1980 when that agency announced that it would remove from the market over ensuing years more than 3,000 drugs whose effectiveness had not been established. It is estimated that Americans spent at least $1 billion on these unproven drugs in 1979 alone.

Ten of the drugs were on the list of the 100 most prescribed medicines in 1979. Among them was Dimetapp, a decongestant that was prescribed nearly 15 million times in 1979 at a cost of about $67 million. The list also included four Phenergan expectorants, which were prescribed 11 million times in 1979 and cost the anxious mothers whose children took them about $52 million.

Now, here's the shocker that you might remember the next time you visit the physician who has been feeding your kids these medicines for all these years: The FDA action to remove

Dimetapp and Phenergan from the market came as the result of a court action filed by two consumer groups. The suit was instituted to force the FDA to implement the drug effectiveness amendments to the Food, Drug, and Cosmetics Act *that were passed by Congress in 1962!*

Those amendments required that manufacturers prove the effectiveness of the drugs they were selling by October 1964. Yet the manufacturers had resisted all efforts to force them to prove that their drugs worked, or remove them from the market, for nearly twenty years. Meanwhile, doctors continued to prescribe them despite the inability of the manufacturers to prove that they were effective in treating the ailments for which they were prescribed.

One must assume that, over those two decades, the drug companies did their utmost to prove that these highly profitable drugs really worked. They didn't succeed, but they kept them on the market anyway. Considering this deplorable eagerness to rip off the public by selling unproven drugs, how much effort do you think the industry spent on research to determine whether the drugs they were selling might actually do harm?

The danger to your health doesn't end even when the drugs you take are effective, safe, and prescribed for the purpose for which they are intended—a happy combination that is not often achieved. In 1973, a study of the prescriptions that doctors ordered and hospital pharmacists filled was done in the pediatric emergency room of a major urban teaching hospital. More than 4,300 prescriptions were written for 2,403 patients by eighteen physicians and filled by nine pharmacists. The results of the study were limited to the seventy most popular drugs, which were prescribed 2,213 times.

Only 5 percent of those prescriptions contained no errors! Residents— with an extra year of training—made more mistakes than interns. Errors included incorrect dosages, incorrect time intervals, incorrect quantities, and inadequate instructions to the patient. Given the inverse ratio of experience and training to accuracy one must wonder whether if the performance of attending staff physicians had been studied their error rate would have been 100 percent!

Why are doctors so casual about dispensing prescriptions for inadequately tested, toxic, potentially dangerous drugs that may do women more harm than good? I can give you several reasons that explain the practice, but none that will help your doctor maintain your trust.

Primary among them is the motive that dominates all Modern Medicine—its dedication to medical intervention and its eagerness to try every new drug that appears on the scene. Second is an abysmal ignorance of the effects of drugs, a subject that gets little attention in medical schools. Third is the economic incentive to prescribe medications, particularly among group practices that have their own pharmacies and profit directly from the prescriptions they write. Finally, most doctors won't spend the time and don't have the inclination to explore the psychological roots of their patients' complaints or provide the kind of sympathetic, compassionate counseling they need. They find it easier and more profitable to get women out of their offices by handing them a prescription for pills.

As a consequence of this attitude, two out of three visits to doctors end with prescriptions. The doctors write them to terminate consultations, not to solve the patients' problems. The patient leaves with the problem that brought her there, plus a prescription that may create new problems that will bring her back again.

The penchant of the medical profession for dispensing drugs at every opportunity comes as no surprise to me, for it is one of the things that I, too, was taught in medical school. During my residency a prominent senior pediatrician told me that I should never send a patient out of the office without a piece of paper in her hand. If not a prescription for a drug, then a diet for her baby or some other instruction—but always put a piece of paper in her hand.

Many patients, of course, believe that there is a drug for every ailment, but only because they have been indoctrinated to believe it by doctors and drug companies. There's more money in peddling pills than in proffering reassurance and sound advice. Yet, when doctors are charged with overmedicating their patients, the typical response is, "the patient wanted it."

This "blame the victim" strategy is one that doctors employ to cover most of their sins, whether the transgression lies in pushing drugs, or performing hysterectomies and Caesarean sections that their patients shouldn't have and don't need.

I've heard this apologia from almost every doctor I know, and each time I marvel at the inconsistency. If doctors find it so difficult to resist the demands of their patients for medications and surgical procedures that earn a lot of money, where do they find the energy and determination to oppose so bitterly any innovative treatment—like chiropractic or nutrition therapies—that they can't provide?

A woman who wants to stay healthy must learn to protect herself from dangerous and unnecessary drugs. Don't expect that your doctor will do it for you. Ask him to show you the prescribing information for every drug that he asks you to take. Pay particular attention to the warnings and notes on side effects. If you don't like what you read, make him defend his use of the drug. If he can't or won't do that, it is time to consider whether you should have a talk with somebody else.

8

"I'm Afraid We'll Have to Operate."

The fact that you are a woman living in the United States greatly reduces the chances that you'll survive to a ripe old age with all of your organs intact. The number of operations performed in America has been increasing steadily and now exceeds 20 million a year. Those performed exclusively on women lead the list.

If all of the surgery performed on American women made you healthier, Modern Medicine would deserve your applause. Unfortunately, it doesn't. Surgeons in this country operate twice as often as those in England and Wales, without any significant difference in therapeutic results! The only thing American women have to show for much of this knifemanship is the world's largest collection of surgical scars.

Men and women do not share the burden of this surgical epidemic equally. In 1977, five of the ten most commonly performed surgical procedures, and more than half of the total operations included in this group, were obstetrical-gynecological.

Modern Medicine would like you to believe that American women are fortunate to receive all of this high-priced attention. The surgeons would have a case if they practiced their wizardry only in cases of genuine need. Too often it is the surgeons, not the patients, who have the need. Dr. John Bunker, a Stanford University researcher who has studied the nation's shocking incidence of surgery confirms what I have long observed. He says that "Not more than 20 percent of surgery is done to prevent death or prolong life. The rest is done to improve the quality of life, and we have no systematic data on the value of the results." In other words, four out of five operations are done because the surgeon says they will make you feel better, but there is no real evidence that they actually do. With more than 16 million operations a year in this category, I believe it is time to demand that the surgeons try to find out.

I'm convinced that women have needless surgery because we have more surgeons than we need. A 1970 study by two of the surgeons' own associations found that the United States already had 22,000 more surgeons than necessary, and the number has been increasing ever since. Clearly the odds are high, and getting higher, that at some time in your life you will become the lawful prey of a surgeon who is looking for work to do. When that happens there are some things you should know before you let him carve you up. There are also some steps you can take to lessen the risk that you will endure an operation that you don't really need.

First, don't assume without further inquiry that the operation is really necessary or that it will do you any good.

The number of needless elective operations performed in this country is a medical disgrace. Studies have repeatedly shown that the amount of surgery performed varies greatly from one locality to another and that this difference is not determined by medical need. Instead, it correlates directly with the presence of surgeons who need surgery to do and with the number of beds that hospitals need to fill.

The manner of payment also affects the amount of surgery

performed. When prepaid plans, in which surgeons are salaried, are compared with fee-for-service plans, the results are startling. Doctors whose income depends on the number of operations they perform do 50 to 100 percent more surgery than those who receive the same salary no matter how many patients they put under the knife.

An even more dramatic example of the extent to which economic incentives determine the performance of surgery was demonstrated two years ago when Blue Cross–Blue Shield decided to stop paying for twenty-eight procedures that were deemed ineffective. When they were no longer covered by insurance, which put a heavier burden on the doctor to justify them to the patient, the incidence of these types of surgery dropped 75 percent almost overnight.

One of these useless procedures was performed exclusively on women whose pelvic ligaments had stretched. Known as the uterine suspension, it was being imposed on about 8,000 female victims each year, and it cost them or their insurance companies $5,000 to $6,000 each. All the patient had to show for the money and the misery was an abdominal scar—hardly a bargain at $1,000 an inch.

Another reason for the greater incidence of surgery in the United States than in Great Britain is the difference in the systems of medical care. Under Britain's National Health Service, surgeons are hospital-based and see only patients who are referred to them by internists and general practitioners. In the United States, surgeons can accept patients without referral. In fact, the surgeon may be the woman's primary physician, often a gynecologist who acts as judge, jury, and sometimes executioner. He diagnoses the ailment, determines whether surgery can be employed, and then performs the operation himself. American surgeons have exhibited considerable ingenuity in creating their own demand, and I doubt that their creativity has been exhausted yet. Surgeons are already performing prophylactic mastectomies, and I anticipate the day when the surgical concept of preventive medicine will consist of removing any portion of the anatomy that might someday get sick.

The evidence is clear: We have too many surgeons who are being paid to do too many operations that their patients don't need. A variation of Parkinson's Law is at work: The number of needless operations performed increases to fill the time of those who are paid to do them.

In 1976, a congressional committee concerned about the soaring costs of medical care studied the problem of unnecessary surgery in the United States. It reported that in 1974, doctors performed nearly 2.4 million unnecessary operations. Think of it! This is about equivalent to placing every resident of Kansas, Colorado, Mississippi, or South Carolina on the operating table for surgery they don't need.

The committee estimated the cost of this worthless surgery at nearly $4 billion. Undoubtedly, it wiped out the life savings of many families, forcing some into bankruptcy or overwhelming debt. Yet those who paid only with money were the "lucky" victims. *About 12,000 patients paid with their lives.*

To put the tragedy of this useless surgery in perspective, consider this: In 1974, knives were the instrument of 15,000 absolutely senseless deaths in the United States. Three thousand of them were used by murderers. In the other 12,000 cases a surgeon held the knife!

Second, don't believe your surgeon if he tells you that the knifemanship he wants to practice on you is "very low risk," or "perfectly safe."

The only completely safe operation is the one you refuse to permit. The spectre of death hangs over *every* surgical procedure. The most obvious and dramatic surgical risks, which turn up in malpractice suits, involve the surgeon's knife that slips and the gear he forgets to remove before he closes you up. In one incredible case a 30-inch towel stamped "U.S. Army" was left behind.

I always counsel my students to go with their patients to surgery, watch the surgeon, and ask him the kinds of questions relatives would ask if they were given the chance. I tell them that if a biopsy is taken, they should go with the specimen to the pathology lab, look in the microscope, and question the pathologist. It is good insurance against surgical overkill or error. If your doctor sends you to a surgeon, I recommend that you ask him to accompany you.

Besides surgical error, and the possibility of getting the wrong operation because you are mixed up with somebody else, the major risk is anesthesia, which can cause death from anaphylactic shock, convulsions, choking on vomit, and cardiac arrest. It can also interfere with the functions of the respiratory system, heart and blood vessels, kidneys, and brain. Anesthesia causes or contributes to death about once in every 3,000 surgical cases. With more than 20 million operations being performed annually in the United States, that comes out to about 7,000 deaths a year. Errors or complications associated with blood transfusions during or after surgery cause another 2,500 deaths a year. The risks of hepatitis increase if paid donors are used, so the cautious woman will ask her doctor about the source of the blood she is given. Finally, all surgery exposes the patient to postoperative complications, some of which result in permanent damage or death. They include pneumonia, blood clots, shock, infection, and hemorrhage.

Mortality rates vary greatly from one type of surgery to another, and you should insist on knowing what they are before you submit to an operation of any kind. The mortality rate for abdominal hysterectomies, for example, is about 1 percent. If a gynecologist tries to talk you into one by assuring you that your chances of dying on the operating table are only one in 100, ask him who will take care of your kids if you end up among the 1 percent.

Third, don't be deceived by the aura of confidence that your surgeon exudes.

It's one of the things they teach in medical school, and even the students who don't learn much else do learn that. It masks their own feelings of insecurity and intimidates everyone else. Because the quality of his performance is never really measured, a doctor doesn't have to be a very good surgeon in order to prosper. He just has to know how to act like one. I suspect, particularly in the case of some of the fancy Park Avenue or Beverly Hills-type specialists, that there may be an inverse ratio between the skill of a doctor and the size of his bank account. Unfortunately, I haven't figured out how to prove it.

Fourth, don't buy your surgeon's assurances about the comfort and security you're going to enjoy in your hospital bed.

I've spent enough years in hospitals to know, despite their antiseptic appearance, that they're the most germ-laden places in town. Hospital patients contract so many germ-induced infections that doctors even have a word for them. We call them nosocomial infections, which enables us to discuss your new ailment in your presence without revealing that you wouldn't have it if you had stayed at home.

Despite the impression created by all those crisp, white uniforms, hospitals aren't all that efficient, either, except in the business office, which is always as efficient as all get out. For one thing, hospitals are prone to handle their laundry so carelessly that those antiseptic-appearing uniforms are often loaded with germs. Not just ordinary germs, either. Hospitals harbor a variety of them that could keep an army of bacteriologists busy for the rest of their lives.

What's inside the uniforms can also leave something to be desired. If you experience a life-threatening emergency while you are hospitalized, you can't assume that your troubles are over when that self-important man in the white coat appears at your side. Not even if he has his badge of office, the stethoscope, hanging around his neck. He may be a medical student or an intern or a first-year resident who hasn't slept for a couple of days, doesn't know what to do but doesn't dare admit it, and is scared stiff that you may expire while he's in charge. Sometimes his lack of experience assures that result.

Most patients assume they are talking to a doctor if he's wearing a white coat, is adorned with a stethoscope, and has a chart in his hand. Often they are not. But the medical students won't correct you when you call them "Doctor," for it's music to their ears. In reality, the students, interns, and residents are the hospital equivalents of Chinese coolies. They work a long and arduous schedule for little or no pay in exchange for the privilege of sharpening their shaky skills on you.

The resident physicians are also there to gain experience and develop their skills at your expense. In at least one respect, they may present a greater risk than the students and the interns. In order to qualify in their specialty, surgical residents must perform certain procedures a specific number of times. The vast majority who are males can't perform Caesarean sections or hysterectomies on each other, so they have to have female patients. If a resident hasn't filled his quota of all the appropriate operations, and you give him half a chance, he is strongly motivated to find an excuse to use one of these surgical procedures on you.

Your closest contact in the hospital will be with the attendants and the nurses. They are abused terribly by the male staff members, but they do the best they can under trying circumstances. Hospital mortality rates would soar if the nurses weren't around to pick up the pieces the doctors leave behind. But in all honesty, as good as they usually are, they are often so harassed and overworked that they make errors, too. And, just as with the doctors, the consequences can be terminal if one of them makes a mistake.

The University of Cincinnati gave a series of test problems to twenty-seven registered nurses in the newborn intensive care unit. The purpose was to determine how accurate they were in calculating the appropriate drug doses for the babies in their care. The nurses gave the right answer less than half the time. *The margin of error in some cases was an incredible 1,000 percent!* With some medications, the overdoses would have been enough to kill the babies if the medicine had actually been given.

It's no real consolation, but the residents and attending physicians who were given the same problem often did no better.

Fifth, don't assume that your surgeon is so well-trained and conscientious that he never makes a mistake.

So much attention has been paid to the high level of academic performance required for admission to medical school and the years of arduous training required to get an M.D., that most people seem to assume that a doctor can do no wrong.

In 1973-75, in a rare example of self-scrutiny, the American College of Surgeons and the American Surgical Association studied nearly 1,500 cases in which patients had complications during or after surgery. The study involved ninety-five hospitals in seven states. They found that *one-third of the deaths and almost half of the complications from surgery could have been prevented.* Surgeon's errors were responsible for an incredible 78 percent of the preventable complications, half of which were from faulty surgical techniques.

Even the hidebound American Medical Association at last discovered in 1980 that doctors aren't perfect. After operating for 133 years on the premise that its members could do no wrong, it finally revised its code of ethics and called for more effective self-policing to weed out unethical and incompetent doctors. Dr. James Todd, of Ridgewood, New Jersey, who headed the code-revision committee, said: "A lot of physicians don't like to concede that there are incompetent doctors. But we all know that there are incompetent people in any profession."

It says something about the institution of medicine that it took one and one-third *centuries* to discover that! But note that the AMA calls for self-policing, and don't hold your breath until you begin to see incompetent doctors actually being weeded out.

Sixth, don't presume that your surgeon has considered less risky and damaging forms of treatment and turned to surgery only as a last resort.

Surgeons are trained to *do* surgery, not to avoid it. They have little enthusiasm for that priceless line by Oliver Wendell Holmes, "Joy, temperance, and repose, slam the door in the doctor's nose." Indeed, they give short shrift to the likely possibility that in many cases time and natural healing processes will cure the problem with no medical intervention at all. If a surgical option is available, they have no incentive to consider the possibility that a healthy diet, rest, and exercise might very well produce an equal or better result. After all, they aren't selling groceries, mattresses, or jogging shoes. They *believe* in surgery, they *like* to do surgery, they *need* to do surgery, and they've been *taught* to do surgery whenever a plausible excuse can be found.

Finally, don't assume that when a surgeon slices open your belly and snips away at your insides it is going to make you feel any better.

It isn't likely that the surgeon will tell you so up front, but the long-term consequences of surgery often may be worse than the disease. But then, the surgeon didn't promise you a rose garden. His contract was to remove your uterus, and you're supposed to feel grateful if he gave you an unexpected bonus and took your ovaries and tubes as well. How that affects the rest of your life is not his problem, because that's not one of the things they taught him to worry much about while he was in medical school. He did what you paid him to do, and he is proud of his "success" if he gets you out of the hospital alive.

In my years of medical practice I've seen a lot of surgery performed because surgeons believe that God blundered mightily when He created the human physique. You're supposed to regard it as providential that they're around to repair God's mistakes.

In later chapters I'll talk about the widespread surgical abuse that is specific to women. Right now, though, I want to alert you to the vulnerability of your appendix, which doctors remove from women far more often than from men.

Most surgeons regard the appendix, which they remove with impunity with little or no indication of infection, as another of God's mistakes. There isn't a shred of evidence to support that claim, but I can't tell you the number of times I have heard a surgeon tell a woman that the appendix is "a useless, vestigial organ"—some of God's leftover physiological junk.

In 1975, 784,000 appendectomies were performed in the United States and about 3,000 of the patients died. Most of them were described as "emergency" operations performed to prevent the appendix from rupturing and causing peritonitis and even death. Yet, one out of four of the appendixes that were removed were found to be perfectly healthy when they reached the pathology lab.

Surgeons rationalize being wrong one-fourth of the time on the basis that it is safer to remove some healthy organs than it is to wait for the appendix to rupture and increase the mortality risk. Some surgeons even advocate removal of appendixes as a preventive measure, "just in case" they may become infected at some time during the patient's life.

In my judgment, that is the height of irresponsibility, if not idiocy. Statistically, your chances of getting appendicitis are about one in twelve, and the mortality rate is 1 to 2 percent, depending on whether it perforates. That makes your chances of dying from appendicitis about one in 1,200 or one in 600 if it perforates. The chances that you will die from an appendectomy are one in 100, so preventive surgery makes absolutely no sense. It's like chopping down the prettiest tree in your yard "before" it gets Dutch elm disease, "just in case" it might.

Beyond the immediate risks of surgery, how will losing your "useless" appendix affect you for the rest of your life? I don't know, and neither do the surgeons, because very little effort has been made to find out. Studies done by one eminent researcher showed that persons whose appendixes had been removed were twice as likely to develop cancer of the bowel. He concluded that the appendix may be important to the body's resistance to all forms of disease.

So, preventive surgery does trouble me, and it should trouble you. Women are more vulnerable than men to what surgeons call an "incidental appendectomy." These occur when the surgeon, in the course of removing your uterus, says to himself, "Well, I'm in here anyway; I might as well zip her appendix out, too."

One researcher became curious about why so many surgeons removed healthy appendixes in the course of other operations. It couldn't be simply because, like Mt. Everest, they were there. He surveyed the directors of approved residencies in general surgery and obstetrics-gynecology in the United States to determine their attitudes toward incidental appendectomies. *Well over 60 percent of them recommended removal of the appendix when uncomplicated hysterectomies are performed.* More than half of the directors of surgery programs recommended them in other types of abdominal operations, as well.

Imagine! These are the men who are teaching the surgeons of the future. No wonder Modern Medicine is so quick to intervene surgically, at the drop of a hat. Surgeons are simply doing what they were taught.

One of the "givens" about surgical practice in the United States is that, given the opportunity, doctors will do what they know how to do. To understand why, you must look behind Modern Medicine's altruistic, benevolent facade and explore the dogmatic, callous, cutthroat educational process that puts the knife in the surgeon's hand.

During my years of teaching I have been saddened and depressed by the metamorphosis that occurs as young men and women struggle to attain their medical degrees. As entering premedical students, they are eager but constantly apprehensive idealists. Then, as the months and years race by, I watch as their nobler instincts erode in the face of the medical profession's common personality trait—fear. Not fear of the bloody, demanding, and hazardous work that doctors must do, but fear that they will never have the chance to do it.

Premedical students know that fifty or sixty candidates will be competing for every opening in medical school, in which only the most aggressive and least-principled students are likely to survive. They soon learn that to make it in the competition they must give blind allegiance to the conventional, self-serving, often indefensible doctrine of the curriculum, to cheat when possible, to undercut their peers when necessary, and to butter up the chief residents and attending staff whenever the opportunity presents itself.

Through their association with the attending surgeons whom they assist, the surgical residents learn other things that are even more damaging. They learn to conceal from the patient the risks and potential side effects that most surgery entails. They learn that doctors cover up each other's mistakes. They learn to "sell" unnecessary or borderline procedures as though they were dealing in used cars. Under all of these pressures, the suffering human beings they once cared about become so many profitable slabs of meat.

My colleagues who head the nation's medical schools boast that this process of "survival of the fittest" assures Americans of the finest medical care in the world. My observation is that doctors are taught to provide a lot of medical and surgical intervention, but I don't see evidence of very much "care." The fittest *do* survive, but what are they fit for? They are the survivors of a heartless system that too often weeds out the best and the bravest—the students with compassion, integrity, intelligence, creativity, and the courage to resist the destruction of their own moral and ethical codes.

Fledgling doctors who have completed surgical residencies have learned all too well that *radical intervention* is the name of the game. Too often the comfort and future well-being of the patient is not the issue; the surgery has become an end in itself.

What can you do to protect yourself when your doctor says you need surgery?

First of all, don't rush home and pack your toothbrush. At least 80 percent of all surgery is elective, which means you *do* have a choice, and there are few occasions in medicine when you have anything to lose by waiting a few days. Obviously, if you are the victim of an honest-to-God life-and-death emergency, the following advice doesn't apply. But if that's what you're faced with, someone else will probably make the decision for you anyway, because you'll be too sick even to hear the siren on the ambulance. If your case is not a genuine emergency, delay your decision and give yourself some time to make up your mind.

Ask a lot of questions, and insist on real answers. Don't let your doctor give you a comforting pat and put you off. What kind of questions? For starters, try these:

Is this surgery really necessary? Insist on a detailed explanation of your condition, what surgery will do to correct it, and what your physical and emotional condition will be in the future as a consequence of the surgery. If the doctor is evasive, see someone else.

What will happen to me if I say, "No"? Find out whether your ailment is life-threatening, or will adversely affect your physical comfort or lifestyle if you don't have the operation. Can the surgeon assure you that the operation will improve your comfort and well-being and will not cause side effects that are as bad or worse?

Are there less costly, less risky alternatives? Have your surgeon explain what all of the alternative forms of treatment are and how their results compare with those of the surgical procedure. Ask him about scientific studies or statistics that back up what he says.

What is the mortality rate from this procedure? You are entitled to know the risks of the surgery your doctor plans to perform. Other than some forms of cancer, for which mortality is calculated on the basis of years of survival, the mortality percentages for most surgery sound quite small. A 1 percent mortality rate doesn't sound particularly threatening, especially to doctors, but why risk it if another form of treatment will afford comparable relief?

*What is **your** mortality rate from this procedure?* This question asks your surgeon to compare his own skill with the average of his peers. If his own rate is in the ball park, he has no reason not to tell you so. If he gets angry and refuses to answer, watch out! Go see someone else.

How many of these operations have you performed? Practice makes perfect. You should pick a surgeon who operates frequently and has had a lot of experience with the operation he plans to perform on you. Some experts say that a surgeon should do at least ten operations a week in order to maintain a high level of skill.

If you had my condition, would you have this surgery? It's a cinch he'll say "Yes." Your task is to sense how sincere he is when he says it.

If you did, who would you have perform it on you? If the answers to your other questions have left you dissatisfied, this one may identify another surgeon to consult.

If I have this surgery, how long will it take me to recover? Determine how long the recovery period will be, how extensively it will limit your activities, and what debilitating long-term side effects it may have that will affect your life, your family, or your job.

How much will this operation cost? Before you go to the hospital you should know the cost of the surgery, the subsequent hospital care, and the cost of the hospitalization itself. Are expensive tests required? What will the anaesthesiologist charge? What is the estimated amount of your hospital bill? How much of this will your insurance cover? If the potential benefits of the surgery are minimal, they may not justify the cost.

Could I delay the operation and try some other form of treatment first? You've already asked this question in different words, but ask again. If he says no, be suspicious. Don't agree to surgery until your doctor has convinced you that there is no alternative treatment that may work. It may be worth trying, unless the delay will make your condition substantially worse.

Asking these questions may also be of value if you do proceed with the surgery and experience negative consequences that your doctor failed to warn you about in advance. Out of the plethora of malpractice suits that have been tried in recent years has emerged a legal doctrine of "informed consent." If your physician fails to inform you fully about the potential risks and side effects of the operation he is about to perform, or if it does not live up to his assurances, or if something avoidable goes wrong, you will be justified in suing your doctor for the damage he has caused. Make careful note of the answers you get to these questions because it is information that you may need if you ultimately decide to sue.

Most Americans hold my profession in so much awe that they are reluctant to ask their doctor questions like these. Don't be. You may wound his vanity, but that's better than being wounded yourself. If you're persistent, he must either answer your questions or throw you out.

In either event, get a second opinion, and if you're still uncertain get a third opinion or as many as you need to make an intelligent choice. Don't get it from someone your first doctor recommends. If Charlie McCarthy said you needed surgery, you'd be an idiot to go to Edgar Bergen for further advice. Don't go to one of your doctor's partners. Don't go to someone on the same hospital staff. And if you really want to protect yourself, go out of town. Go anywhere you have to go to get the best, most honest advice. When I made that recommendation on the Phil Donahue show, Donahue remarked, "You've got to have a real, real good American Express card to do all this." That's true, but many insurance policies will now pay for a second opinion; some even require it. That's because they have discovered that when a second opinion is sought, half the proposed operations are never performed.

In any event, the return on your investment in a second opinion may be the kind that would make a stockbroker beam. A coronary bypass operation costs between $12,000 and $20,000, and surgeons have been performing them like they were kids with a new toy. They don't tell you about the studies that show that those who have the bypass and those who don't experience about the same results. Second opinions do cost money, but you could afford to travel around the world to get one if it saved you the agony of surgery and $20,000.

Wherever you go for your second opinion, make sure that the consultant you choose understands that all you want from him is advice. It's important for him to know that if he recommends surgery, he won't be the one who does the work.

Don't reveal to the consultant the advice that you have already received. Have him do his own workup, and if the first surgery was recommended on the basis of laboratory tests, have them done over again. Medical laboratories are notoriously inaccurate, and it is folly to make a judgment based on one set of test results. If x-rays were involved, ask your doctor to let you take them with you. There is no point in exposing yourself to some more dangerous radiation if you don't have to. But you do want to have them read by another radiologist to be sure that the first one read them right. There is ample evidence that two radiologists reading the same set of x-rays will disagree with each other. In fact, as noted earlier, a radiologist reading a set of x-rays for a second time will often disagree with himself!

If the surgery is elective, as most surgery is, and your doctor is vague about the side effects and the potential impact of the operation on the future quality of your life, check with others who have survived the same procedure. Go to the library and look it up in some books. You may discover that you'd rather live with the ailment than with the side effects of the cure.

Avoid teaching hospitals if you decide that you must have the surgery. That statement defies the conventional wisdom, but I've spent a lot of time in teaching hospitals and I think it is good advice. Teaching hospitals are exactly what the name implies. They are hospitals that exist so that students can learn. Enter one, and they'll get their on-the-job training practicing on you. Obviously, there is a point at which every surgical resident must take his first slice at a nice, warm belly, but do you really want it to be the one that belongs to you?

Depending on the nature of your problem, don't hesitate to consult practitioners who are not welcome in Modern Medicine's hallowed halls. Doctors are always warning their patients about the dangers of consulting "medical quacks" or resorting to "unscientific, unproven remedies." Meanwhile, they have made a living dispensing therapy from their own bag of unproven, unscientific, and often worthless "cures."

Until 1980, the American Medical Association's code of ethics prevented a licensed physician from recommending or even associating with a chiropractor because his method of healing was not "founded on a scientific basis." Increasingly, however, this position was subjected to legal challenges, and suddenly the AMA found itself spending three-quarters of a million dollars a year defending itself in suits. Worse, if the AMA lost the suits then pending, it could have been bankrupted.

Nothing had happened that suddenly made chiropractic less threatening to its patients, but it had become a threat to the survival of the AMA. The old ban was dropped, and doctors are now free to refer patients to chiropractors, acupuncture specialists, herbalists, faith healers, and others who operate on the fringes of medical science.

I find this fascinating because I recall, when I was a medical student more than thirty years ago, being warned not to consort with chiropractors. Later, social contact with them became acceptable, although not encouraged, but consultation was still taboo. Now, with the 1980 change in the AMA ethics code, I am allowed to refer patients to chiropractors and receive patients from them.

Now that the ban on consultation has been lifted, I can predict what will happen next. Modern Medicine will try to co-opt chiropractic, as it has other therapeutic methods, such as osteopathy, that it once labeled "quack." If it accomplishes that, the new "science" of chiropractic will be surrounded with a vocabulary of medical mumbo-jumbo, and a board will be established to certify chiropractic specialists, making it impossible for anyone to become a chiropractor who hasn't been brainwashed in one of the establishment's captive medical schools.

So, if you have an ailment that it is appropriate for him to treat, don't feel sheepish about seeing a chiropractor. I have seen more than one case in which spinal surgery was avoided by individuals who decided, as a last resort before going under the knife, to see a chiropractor about their aching backs.

If you suspect that diet may have something to do with your problem, see a nutritional authority. Most doctors don't know anything about nutrition, because medical schools are so oriented toward intervention that they virtually ignore nutrition as an element in the prevention or cure of disease. If you are concerned about something related to childbearing or gynecology, I'd even recommend consulting a couple of grandmothers. Compared with some obstetricians I know, they make much more sense.

Inevitably, surgery is most often recommended when you are in the most vulnerable psychological and emotional condition. You're sick, worried, frightened, and probably overwrought. It is the worst possible time to be confronted with a decision that could mean your life.

It may not be easy, but hang on to your wits. However imposing your surgeon's credentials are, and however commanding his presence may be, don't take what he tells you at face value. He has been taught to do surgery, he believes in it as the cure for all ills, and when confronted by a set of symptoms, surgery is what he will almost always want to do.

Your challenge is to decide whether you ought to let him do it to you.

9

"What Do You Need a Uterus for, Anyway?"

It is appalling to contemplate, but if Modern Medicine continues on its present course *one of every two women in the country will part with her uterus before she reaches the age of 65.*

American surgeons performed about 690,000 hysterectomies in 1979. It is doubtful that more than one in five of them could be justified as clinically necessary on the basis of life-threatening medical needs. That means that more than half a million endured the operation for reasons that were frivolous at worst and dubious at best.

The hazards of this indiscriminate surgery are so alarming that they prompted a congressional investigation in 1977. Predictably, the principal spokesman for the American Medical Association rose to the surgeons' defense. Dr. James H. Sammons, executive vice-president of the AMA, invoked Modern Medicine's standard "blame the victim" strategy. The increase in hysterectomies, he said, was due to their elective use as a "convenient form of sterilization" and to their prophylactic use to eliminate the possibility of uterine cancer in future years. He asserted that, while the surgery could not be considered "clinically necessary" for either of these reasons, it was beneficial to women with excessive anxiety, "and therefore necessary."

As his clincher, Dr. Sammons asserted that the hysterectomy rate among doctors' wives is greater than it is for other women, which presumably justified the high rate at which they are being performed. Regrettably, no one on the committee thought to ask him whether any surveys have been done on how doctors feel about their wives!

As far as I'm concerned, Dr. Sammons' espousal of hysterectomy for the relief of anxiety is indistinguishable from the archaic medical view of the uterus as the seat of hysteria. To put the sexism of this argument in perspective, you need only apply the same principle to a male patient who is experiencing anxiety because of a morbid fear that he may develop cancer of the penis. How many male surgeons would "cure" his anxiety by cutting it off?

The use of hysterectomies for prophylactic purposes is akin to getting rid of mice by setting fire to the house. There are less hazardous ways to prevent conception, and removal of the uterus to prevent cancer makes no sense at all. There is less chance that a woman will die from uterine cancer than that she will die when a hysterectomy is performed. Once again, the disease is less deadly than Modern Medicine's cure.

When I confront a gynecologist with the staggering rise in the hysterectomy rate he almost always responds with the "blame the victim" excuse. It is remarkable how pliable doctors claim to be in the hands of their female patients when the result is income from non-diseases that they can treat. To hear them tell it, they simply can't resist when patients plead for surgery they don't need. Besides, the doctors maintain, it wouldn't do any good to say "No," because their patients would shop for another surgeon who is willing to do the job.

It's a convenient argument, but it is harder to swallow than a handful of pills. If anyone seeks, much less shops for, a hysterectomy, it is because she has not been adequately informed of the hazards and consequences of the surgery. I don't believe that "popular demand" will explain away the fact that the United States has the highest hysterectomy rate in the world—two and one-half times that of England, and four times that of Sweden and some other European countries. A more reasonable explanation is the fact that those countries have state-paid health plans that remove the economic incentive to perform more surgery.

At one time hysterectomies were performed mainly when cancer was present—a life-threatening situation. Today, only about 20 percent are performed because of indications of cancer. One-third are done because of the presence of benign fibroid tumors on the inside walls of the uterus. One out of every four women over age twenty-five has such tumors, but most of them cause no trouble and disappear with the onset of menopause. Unless there are symptomatic problems because of these tumors—severe pain or bleeding, for example—there is no medical justification for removing the uterus.

Many hysterectomies have been performed to correct over-stretched pelvic ligaments—a condition known as *slipped uterus*. I wonder how many women would agree to surgery for this condition if they were told of an often adequate alternative—a good girdle! Even more incredible are the hysterectomies that have been performed as a treatment for migraine headaches, which probably also are traceable to the Dark Age perception of female emotions. No less an authority than the late Dr. Walter Alvarez, of the Mayo School of Medicine, once reported knowledge of at least 100 such cases, none of which could be justified on the basis of any scientific evidence that the surgery would do any good.

There is only one rational explanation for all of the needless hysterectomies that are being performed. Doctors, being dedicated to the most extreme forms of intervention and wanting the income that comes from intervening, fail their patients miserably by not giving them the information they need in order to make an informed choice.

How many women would permit, much less seek, a hysterectomy for a reason that was not life-threatening if they knew that in 1975 more than 1,100 women died from the procedure? How many would welcome sharing the misery experienced by more than 30 percent of the patients who had some type of infection as a result of the surgery, or the one in six who required blood transfusions? How many women would relish being exposed to the additional danger of infectious hepatitis from the transfused blood or from the equipment used in delivering intravenous fluids?

Would women deliberately choose hysterectomy as a means of sterilization if they were told that the procedure is twenty times more likely to kill them than is a tubal ligation? Would they accept a hysterectomy as a means of preventing cancer if it were suggested that this was also a good reason to have both breasts removed?

If there were no valid clinical reason for doing it, would women permit the removal of their ovaries and tubes? Many gynecologists do this routinely when they perform a hysterectomy, apparently caring little that their patient will then suffer the rigors of premature menopause. They rationalize this indiscriminate butchery as cancer prevention, despite scientific evidence that it has no value in forestalling that dreaded disease. A study reported in 1977 reviewed more than 2,000 patients who had hysterectomies between 1948 and 1975. The ovaries were retained in more than half of the patients, and most of them benefited because they retained ovarian function until they reached natural menopause. Only fourteen of those patients subsequently required further gynecologic surgery. Only two of them died of cancer, and a review of their cases indicated that they, too, would have survived if they had submitted to periodic followups. In short, none of the patients who retained their ovaries and tubes would have benefited if they had been removed.

How many women who are attracted to hysterectomy as an alternative form of birth control, or to eliminate the nuisance of menstruation, have been led to believe that it is a safe and uncomplicated procedure? Although not one of the most hazardous procedures, it still presents significant risks. Even good surgeons sometimes miscalculate and make mistakes. When they do, unwanted complications crop up, the ultimate of which is death.

Dr. Leroy R. Weeks, a professor of obstetrics-gynecology at the University of Southern California School of Medicine, said in a 1977 study published in the AMA *Journal* that "Complications of gynecological surgery are considerable and when reviewed in detail are almost frightening. . . ." He listed the ten most common errors made by surgeons performing abdominal hysterectomies and concluded:

> Every surgeon has his favorite operation, technique, maxims, and superstitions, and as long as they are being used in the best interest of the patient, all is well. The risk is that he may lose flexibility, *assume a posture of God,* and become careless about the application of his expertise. (Italics added.)

Dr. Weeks's concern extends to all forms of surgery, of course, but women should be informed that in one respect the hazards may be greater in the case of hysterectomies. Many of them are performed by gynecologists who are less qualified than the patient has the right to expect or may believe. In 1975, only 16,000 of the 22,500 physicians who were practicing gynecology were board-certified. The physicians who were not board-certified—presumably the least qualified surgeons—performed hysterectomies three times as often as those who were!

All of the facts about posthysterectomy depression and other psychological complications are rarely given to patients in advance of surgery. Too often, gynecologists sidestep questions about these consequences by assuring women that those that appear can be dealt with by administering estrogen replacements. This is often not true, and, in fact, the patient may suffer additional damage from the cure.

In some of the groups that have been studied carefully, posthysterectomy depression has been experienced by one-third to one-half of the patients. It occurs so frequently that some doctors recommend psychiatric consultation before the surgery is performed on women under age forty-five. The common belief, even among doctors, is that these aftereffects are associated with the premature menopause induced when the ovaries and tubes are taken along with the uterus. This is true, but there is also evidence that these effects may occur even when the tubes and ovaries are left intact. The removal of the uterus itself appears to have an acute effect on ovarian hormone production in some women, and headache, dizziness, hot flashes, depression, and insomnia can be produced by hysterectomy, even when the ovaries are left alone.

A woman who is a professor of psychiatry at the Northwestern University Medical School has conducted studies that noted all of these adverse effects of hysterectomies. Because she is a woman and a behavioral psychologist, Dr. Niles Newton explored another consequence of hysterectomy that may not be important to male gynecologists but certainly is to their patients: the supression of libido following the surgery.

Gynecologists are fond of emphasizing the enhanced sexual pleasure enjoyed by women who have had hysterectomies. This alleged benefit is attributed to the fact that they no longer need fear pregnancy. I have always been suspicious of this claim, although there is no doubt that it may be valid in some cases. However, Dr. Newton's studies have found *reduced sexual drive in 60 percent of the women who have had their uterus and both ovaries removed.* Others have reported that after hysterectomy from 20 to 42 percent of the women studied abstained from sexual intercourse altogether.

I have long suspected that much of the sexual dysfunction that propels women to psychiatrists and marriage clinics is a direct result of hysterectomy. Initially, my suspicion was aroused by the many heartrending letters I have received from women whose sex lives were ruined by the operation. Here are a couple of examples:

Dear Dr. Mendelsohn:

In 1971, I had a complete hysterectomy. About three months later, my husband told me I was no longer a woman and could never satisfy him again. Of course, he apologized later, but I was unable to forget what he said.

I am now forty and he is forty-three. I take hormone pills, but ever since my surgery, intercourse has been painful for me, and I never reach a climax. The doctors I've seen tell me the problem is all in my mind.

My husband is a good man and a good provider, but when it comes to sex, he's a different person than he was before my hysterectomy. Is my condition normal? I'm a miserable person in need of help, and I don't know where to get it.

Dear Doctor:

I had a complete hysterectomy when I was in my thirties. If I had it to do over again, I would never have one. I went to several doctors before I consented to the surgery, and they all agreed the surgery had to be done and that hormones would take care of any subsequent problems I might have. The surgery not only wrecked my sex life, but also ruined my nerves. We had a good sex life before surgery, but now it gets worse each year. It's a bitter pill to swallow when you know you're a failure, and your husband tells you that you're a poor sex partner. The harder I try the worse things get. . . .

I will have to confess that I didn't have a good answer for either of these women or for hundreds of others who have written to me. My hope is that through what I have written in this chapter I will encourage more women to consider the hazards very carefully before they allow themselves to be talked into an elective, medically unnecessary hysterectomy.

I say "talked into" advisedly, because I believe that even those women who welcome hysterectomies do so because they have been conditioned to the idea by their doctors. Women who visit gynecologists to obtain tubal ligations are particularly vulnerable to a variation of the "bait and switch" technique employed by some appliance merchants. In the course of the preoperative examination, the gynecologist finds some minor fibroids in the uterus, which he identifies as tumors. He knows that this immediately conjures up the fear of cancer in the woman's mind. Without actually deceiving her, he then plays on her emotional reaction to the tumors inside her and urges that she solve two problems at once by having a hysterectomy rather than a tubal ligation.

This happens frequently in teaching hospitals, where residents need to perform hysterectomies as part of their training. But gynecologists in private practice also have a strong motivation to substitute hysterectomies for tubal ligations because, at the very least, it will triple their fee.

That the economic motive is strong is demonstrated by the fact that the number of hysterectomies performed on insured patients is double the number performed on the uninsured. In prepaid health plans, where needless surgery is discouraged by peer review, the hysterectomy rates are one-fourth less common than in fee-for-service plans like Blue Cross–Blue Shield.

An increasing supply of gynecological surgeons, coupled with a declining birth rate, has made it more difficult for obstetrician-gynecologists to prosper. The situation can only get worse as surplus doctors pour out of the medical schools during the decade ahead. Without enough patients to go around, gynecologists will be tempted to extract more income from those that they already have by recommending surgery that the patient doesn't really need. Back in 1975, in a *New York Times* interview, a Baltimore specialist frankly admitted that it was already happening: "Some of us aren't making a living, so out comes a uterus or two each month to pay the rent."

Patients in charity hospitals are particularly vulnerable to hysterectomies performed for sterilization. The motive here is also economic, but it comes under the heading of social engineering rather than of personal gain. When the mother has entered labor, the resident physician who is attending says, "You don't really want to have another baby, do you?" At that point she probably doesn't even want the one she is about to have, so she says no. He then persuades her to undergo a hysterectomy. His motive is to gain the experience of doing the hysterectomy, at the same time relieving society of any future welfare costs that would be sustained if the patient had more babies. In some charity hospitals so many hysterectomies are performed on indigent black patients that they are laughingly referred to as *Mississippi appendectomies.* According to one report, surgery performed under these conditions accounts for 10 percent of all gynecologic surgery in New York City.

When the lining of the uterus is afflicted with endometrial cancer, or when other cancers are present in the reproductive system, a hysterectomy may be justified despite the hazards and the potential aftereffects associated with surgical menopause. In the absence of such life-threatening conditions, however, every woman must consider carefully whether the risks of hysterectomy are a sensible trade-off for the dubious benefits that may be realized. Your doctor may try to persuade you that other forms of contraception are inconvenient and less reliable and that menstruation is an unnecessary nuisance, and you may well agree. But that's not really the question. The question you must ask yourself is, are these inconveniences less acceptable than the oppressive symptoms of menopause, psychiatric problems, sexual dysfunction, and the ultimate penalty—death?

Don't accept the assurances of a gynecologist that the menopausal symptoms can be managed by using estrogens such as Premarin. They *can't* always be managed with estrogens, and the estrogens themselves expose the patient to a new set of risks. Studies have established a clear link between estrogen treatment and endometrial cancer. That is of great concern to a woman who undergoes natural menopause but not, of course, to one experiencing posthysterectomy menopause, because her uterus is no longer intact. Of concern to her, however, is the possibility of increased risk of cancer of the breast.

A number of scientific studies have associated the use of estrogen therapy with an increased incidence of cancer of the breast. No responsible authority has yet been willing to state positively that estrogens *cause* cancer of the breast, nor has any responsible authority been able to prove that they don't. Given the possibility that estrogens may be causing breast cancer, you would suppose that doctors would stop prescribing them until the question is resolved. Instead, they continue to observe the ridiculous and deadly principle that drugs are innocent until proven guilty beyond a shadow of a doubt.

Ayerst Laboratories, the manufacturer of Premarin, warns doctors about the risks of endometrial cancer and the use of Premarin during pregnancy in the fine print of its ads in the AMA *Journal,* which few of those who take the drug ever see. The ad also includes this warning: "At the present time there is no satisfactory evidence that estrogens given to postmenopausal women increase the risk of cancer of the breast, although a recent study has raised this possibility."

The caption on the Premarin ad, superimposed over a photograph of a forlorn-looking woman, reads: *The Menopause: Does she have to live with it?*

As one of the physicians to whom the ad is addressed, I'll answer that question.

Isn't it better to learn to live with it than to take their pills and die from them, instead?

10

"It's *You* Your Husband Loves, Not Your Breasts."

Most surgeons, constitutionally flat-chested, can't comprehend the trauma they cause when they chop off a woman's breasts. The scenario that follows their diagnosis too often goes like this:

Mrs. Jones, who is conscientious about doing the things that are necessary to maintain her physical health, wakes up one morning and conducts a self-examination of her breasts. To her dismay, she discovers a small lump in one of them. She visits her gynecologist, who palpates the lump, nods solemnly, and refers her to a surgeon who will perform a biopsy to determine whether the tumor is malignant or benign.

Mrs. Jones is worried, of course, although like most of us, she is prone to thinking of disaster as something that happens to someone else. When she visits the surgeon he reinforces her hope by assuring her that the lump is probably a benign cyst but suggests that she enter the hospital the following week for a biopsy, just to make sure.

The surgeon doesn't tell her about the needle biopsy that could be performed in his office, without the need for a costly hospital stay. He also has her sign a release that authorizes him to perform the biopsy *and any other surgery he feels may be required.* There is no discussion of the alternatives that are available if the lump is diagnosed as a malignant tumor, or of the consequences to Mrs. Jones if he decides to remove the breast if cancer is found.

Mrs. Jones is wheeled into the operating room believing that she is to have a biopsy and nothing more, and hoping against hope that no cancer will be found. When she wakes up in the recovery room she instinctively reaches for her breast and finds that it is gone. Faced with this awful reality she pleads with the nurses for information that they are not permitted to give. She spends hours in the hostile environment of the recovery room, alone with her misery, and without a comforting word from her surgeon, who is nowhere to be found.

Mastectomy is a terribly traumatic experience, even when the woman who endures it is prepared for the loss. The surgeon who inflicts one on a patient without honest discussion of the alternatives, and without advance warning or preparation, may be guilty of the worst mistreatment of all.

Most male surgeons distance themselves from their patients and display little interest in or sympathy for the traumatic reaction of female patients to the loss of one or both breasts. I have no doubt that they would dispute that statement vigorously, but how else can they explain the fact that they still perform radical surgery when the results are no better than other, more desirable procedures?

Many surgeons still perform the horribly disfiguring and debilitating Halsted radical mastectomy, despite overwhelming evidence that it provides no improvement in survival rates over less radical procedures. The extent to which this is determined by lack of empathy for female patients, or dogged devotion to a procedure that was standard treatment for nearly 100 years, can't be measured, but I suspect it is both. Certainly, there is no doubt about the sexist component. One study found that in

Leningrad, where most breast surgery is done by men, the Halsted radical is most commonly used. The modified radical is the preferred procedure in Moscow, where most of the breast cancer surgeons are women.

It is difficult, even for another woman, to appreciate how traumatizing mastectomy is for women who are victims of treatment that was more radical and disfiguring than necessary, or of false biopsy reports done hastily on the operating table that led to surgery that wasn't needed at all. Both of these tragedies occur far more often than you might think.

In October 1980, a New York jury awarded $2.7 million to the family of a woman who lost both breasts because cancer was erroneously diagnosed in biopsy reports. There was nothing humorous about what happened to her, but the testimony about how it happened was almost a comic charade.

The erroneous biopsy reports bore the typewritten name of the assistant to the hospital's chief of pathology, but were unsigned, and he denied any knowledge of them. The chief of pathology, absent when the report was prepared, checked the biopsy specimens on his return. He found no evidence of cancer, and testified that he had so informed the surgeon before the breasts were removed. The surgeon maintained that the operation had been completed before he was informed.

Only one disputed fact emerged from all of the buck-passing. The hapless patient needlessly lost both breasts. She didn't even have the satisfaction of receiving the compensation for her loss, because she died during the seven years that it took for the case to move through the courts.

Shocking, you say? Of course. But in the hallowed halls of Modern Medicine, nothing to get very excited about. It happens all the time, and far more often than the surgeons are forced to admit.

In late 1973, the National Cancer Institute (NCI) and the American Cancer Society (ACS) launched a national cancer detection project in which about 280,000 women began receiving regular mammography examinations at twenty-seven cancer detection centers. By 1976, this massive x-ray screening project had detected about 1,800 cancers. On the surface, this was encouraging evidence of its success. At that point, however, a review was made of the results. *It disclosed forty-eight cases of mistaken diagnosis, thirty-seven of which had resulted in the needless removal of breasts.*

Remember that these examinations were conducted under the auspices of a federal agency and were subjected to a publicized, impartial review. Only the Lord knows how many false biopsies are produced in hospitals and how many women lose their breasts as a result. The only check is an unpublicized postoperative pathology report reviewed by the hospital tissue committee. For the most part, these reviews are so meaningless that some of us now call those who do them "tissue paper" committees, instead.

I have been warning women for years that annual mammographic screening of women without symptoms may produce more cancer than it detects. I haven't been alone. Dr. John C. Bailar III, editor-in-chief of the *Journal of the National Cancer Institute,* made the same point in a 1975 report. His conclusion was supported by numerous studies, which suggested that accumulated x-ray doses in excess of 100 rads over ten to fifteen years may induce cancer of the breast. Dr. Irwin Bross, of the Roswell Park Memorial Institute in Buffalo, New York, also warned a congressional subcommittee in 1978 that the quarter of a million women screened in the NCI-ACS mass screening program will "in fifteen or twenty years become the victims of the worst iatrogenic (doctor-caused) breast cancer epidemic in medical history.

"The big-science federal agencies, their industrial constituencies, and their allies in the engineering, scientific, and medical communities have been lying to the public about the hazards of low-level ionizing radiation for twenty-five years," Dr. Bross said. He added that researchers were rewarded for not finding hazards and punished if they failed to find that low levels of radiation are harmless.

I'm pleased that the NCI and the ACS have finally abandoned routine mammography for women under the age of 50.

Unfortunately, some doctors don't read anything but their bank statements, and still do it nonetheless. Like all x-ray procedures, mammography is potentially dangerous to your health. Unless there are convincing symptomatic reasons for doing one, don't let your doctor do it to you.

Of greater concern to every woman is the continuing penchant of my colleagues in medicine to resort to the most radical form of intervention when confronted by any disease. Nowhere are the consequences of this compulsion more distressing than where breast cancer is concerned.

For nearly a century the Halsted radical mastectomy has been the treatment of choice for most surgeons when breast cancer is diagnosed. The procedure was developed by Dr. William S. Halsted in 1882 and *accepted as standard treatment after the surgery had been demonstrated on only fifty breast cancer victims.* It is defended and routinely used by many surgeons to this very day.

The operation was developed during a period when breast cancers were detected at a much later stage. Consequently, the tumors were usually very large, and often the lymph nodes were clearly involved. Halsted's remedy was to remove the entire breast, the lymph nodes, and the pectoral muscles as well.

Given the state of medical and surgical knowledge a century ago, it is difficult to fault Halsted's reasoning, but that rationalization is no longer valid and hasn't been for many, many years. The operation is an incredibly brutal one, horribly disfiguring and debilitating, as well. It often causes dreadful swelling of the arm and severely limits its use. The cosmetic implications frequently evoke significant psychological reactions in the women who endure the surgery.

Studies have shown that one-fourth of the married women who have mastectomies experience subsequent depression so intense that they have suicidal inclinations. Another quarter experience a deteriorated sexual relationship with their husbands. More than half are victims of *phantom breast syndrome,* a frustrating sensation of feeling in a breast that is no longer there. Psychologists who have studied these reactions blame most of them on inadequate emotional support from the men who performed the operations and from the husbands of the women on whom the surgery was performed.

It is shocking, in view of the devastating nature of this surgical procedure, that it took almost ninety years before the first controlled study of alternatives was conducted. Although other studies had indicated that the survival rate of those who had Halsted radicals was no better than those produced by less radical procedures, the Halsted was almost universally used. Finally, in 1970, the National Cancer Institute sponsored a study of 1,700 women at thirty-four medical centers. It compared three procedures—the radical mastectomy, the simple mastectomy, and the simple mastectomy followed by radiation therapy. The results, in terms of recurrence of the cancer, were virtually the same.

Other scientific studies and clinical trials, here and abroad—at least ten in all—have found no significant differences in survival rates for the various procedures. One of the most recent was conducted by a team of specialists in Rockford, Illinois. They surveyed all the women in that city who had been operated on for breast cancer between 1924 and 1972, whose cases could be followed for at least five years. Most of them could be followed for ten years. After analyzing 1,686 operations they found "no statistically significant differences in five- and ten-year survival for simple, modified radical, and radical mastectomy."

The consensus of those with open minds about the various surgical and radiological alternatives is that survival rates are determined more by the nature of the cancer than by the procedure that is used to treat it. Unfortunately, an open mind is not one of the more striking attributes of many breast surgeons. If it were, more of them would know and act on the fact that mortality from breast cancer typically results from distant metastases of the cancer to other organs, and not from the malignancy of the breast itself.

To put it another way, mortality rates are largely predetermined by factors other than the control of cancer cells in the breast and surrounding tissue. It isn't very comforting to know it, but this is one of those good-news-and-bad-news situations. Patients either have a type of cancer that is confined to the breasts or one that spreads throughout the body. The first type can be cured by local excision of the principal tumor and surrounding tissue, plus radiation of any remaining lesser cancer cells. The type of cancer that metastasizes has usually spread to other parts of the body by the time the disease in the breast is identified, and no form of breast surgery is likely to effect a cure. Although recurrences of cancer in the breast may be somewhat more frequent with the less radical procedures, they can be dealt with readily, without an increase in mortality. I think that most women would rather undergo two non-disfiguring procedures than one procedure that involves loss of a breast.

Knowledge about the current state of the art in breast cancer treatment was summarized in 1979 in a landmark article published in the *Journal of the American Medical Association.* On the basis of careful studies carried out at the Harvard School of Public Health, Dr. Maurice S. Fox, a biologist, reached a number of conclusions that should bring down the curtain on most radical breast surgery. However, if the dedicated radical interventionists in Modern Medicine run true to form, that probably won't happen. His conclusions follow, and I urge you not to forget them, because if the need arises you may want to show your physician or surgeon this page in the book:

1. Radical mastectomy offers no greater benefit than simple mastectomy followed by x-ray therapy.

2. The incidence of diagnosed breast cancer showed an 18 percent increase between 1935 and 1965, and a 50 percent increase between 1965 and 1975. Yet the mortality rate in breast cancer has remained unchanged for at least the last forty years.

3. There appear to be two almost equally divided basic

classes of women with breast cancer; about 40 percent die regardless of the treatment, and the other 60 percent show mortality rates little different from those of women without cancer.

4. Some cancers appear malignant under the microscope but, as far as the patient is concerned, behave in a relatively benign fashion.

5. Although nearly all patients with breast cancer are treated one way or another, those who die rapidly show a mortality rate similar to untreated patients in the nineteenth century.

6. Careful studies of groups of women screened for breast cancer versus similar groups who went unscreened show that the reduction in breast cancer mortality in the first group is not substantially different from the reduction in general mortality exhibited by that group. Furthermore, the group that refused to be screened experienced both a lower incidence of breast cancer and a substantially lower mortality from breast cancer.

7. The striking acceleration of the incidence of diagnosed breast cancer, beginning around 1965, presumably reflects the increasing detection of early disease. Nevertheless, there is no evidence of benefit of this early detection in terms of breast cancer mortality, even ten years later.

8. "It remains possible that much of the occult or early disease detected by screening would never manifest itself as malignant disease in a normal lifetime," Dr. Fox said. "My interpretation of the existing evidence raises questions regarding the wisdom of routine periodic surveys of asymptomatic women."

Dr. Fox's conclusions point up two arguments that I have been making for years. Routine examinations of any kind are dangerous, and mammography is particularly so because it can cause the disease it is used to detect. Second, once any symptom is detected, what can be done will be done, and usually the doctor will select the most radical means. Both of these hazards are compounded by the comparative simplicity of mastectomy. From the surgeon's point of view, breasts—like tonsils—are delightfully easy to get at.

With all of the accumulated evidence that no form of treatment for breast cancer has an appreciable effect on the mortality rate, it would seem prudent that more research be aimed at its causes rather than at unproductive treatments. Since doctors have little or no motivation to look for ways of preventing disease, there is no point in looking to the medical profession for this kind of effort. I think it is time for women to begin making their voices heard—to begin putting some heat on the federal agencies that fund cancer research. I'm convinced that research on the causes of cancer would prove that doctors have been much more successful at producing the disease than they have been at lowering the mortality rate.

My teaching appointment is in the field of preventive medicine, so I have a particular interest in trying to persuade my students to give more attention to the prevention of disease than I find among some of my peers. One of my tricks is to give them a project on how to *produce* disease. My rationale is that if they seriously study what causes diseases, they will pick up some clues on how Modern Medicine must change its behavior in order to prevent it.

In the course of presenting this assignment, I provide the example of how a doctor can produce cancer of the breast. These methods, all of which are already being employed by Modern Medicine and its allies in the pharmaceutical industry, are as follows:

1. Give women the Pill, which studies have linked to cancer of the breast.

2. Prescribe diethylstilbestrol (DES) to dry up breast milk, or as a "morning after" contraceptive pill. If you are able

to give it to a patient who is pregnant, you may get a bonus. It might some day produce cancer in her offspring, too.

3. Discourage your patients from getting pregnant, or perform some surgical wizardry to make sure it doesn't happen. At the very least, try to keep them from making a habit of it, because the more pregnancies a woman has, the less likely it appears that she will develop cancer of the breast.

4. Perform a lot of hysterectomies, and when your patients complain about the menopausal symptoms, keep them on conjugated estrogens for years and years.

5. Discourage breast-feeding whenever possible. It seems to forestall breast cancer. The infant formula manufacturers are generous with samples and will be glad to help.

6. Make sure your patients pick up 100 Rads or so of radiation by x-raying them regularly over the next ten or fifteen years. If you can't find enough excuses to send them for x-rays, get their dentists into the act, or turn up the radiation dosage on the machines.

I can't prove conclusively that any one of these actions will produce breast cancer, but there is so much evidence to support the probability that the ball shouldn't be in my court. If Modern Medicine really cares about the patients it treats, it shouldn't continue to use questionable drugs and procedures until there is proof that they *do* kill people; it should be refusing to use them until there is proof that they don't.

For example, I can't get much attention within the profession for my contention that lactation acts to reduce the incidence of cancer of the breast among nursing mothers. Admittedly, definitive controlled studies are not available to establish an inverse ratio between cancer and breast-feeding beyond a shadow of a doubt. However, I do believe that obstetricians and pediatricians should abandon their role as glorified infant formula salesmen long enough to find out.

In the absence of any scientific interest on their part, I would like them to explain why a 1977 study of Tanka boat women, who traditionally breast-feed only from the right breast, have a higher incidence of cancer in the unsuckled left breast. I would like them to explain why there is a higher incidence of breast cancer among nuns. I'd like to hear them rationalize why a survey of a group of Canadian Eskimo women who traditionally engage in long-term breast-feeding found only one case of breast cancer in a population that ranged from 9,000 to 15,000 over fifteen years. Finally, I'd like to hear their response to a 1964 study at the respected Roswell Park Memorial Institute which found that breast-feeding for seventeen months reduced the risk of breast cancer and that the reduction was even greater when breast-feeding persisted for thirty-six months.

Now that I have explained what women have to fear from Modern Medicine when breast cancer is diagnosed, a legitimate question remains: What do you do when you wake up one morning, conduct a self-examination, and discover a lump in one of your breasts?

First of all, don't panic. The odds are greatly in your favor that the lump you have discovered is benign. Or, even if it is malignant, the chances are good that it can be treated successfully by simple excision and radiotherapy. Your job is to make sure that if that is all you need, that is all you get.

The first step is to obtain a diagnosis from someone you can trust. You don't know anyone you can trust? Then ask around—particularly among other women who have had the same problem—until you have identified two or three of the best specialists in town. Visit each one, tell him what you have discovered, and ask him what he advises you to do.

Hopefully, you will find a surgeon who knows how to do a needle biopsy procedure in his office rather than the more elaborate surgical biopsy procedure that requires admission to a hospital. If all of the surgeons you consult insist that a needle biopsy is inadequate in your case, you may have to accept the more elaborate biopsy procedure. In that event, don't under any circumstances sign a release that will permit the surgeon to remove your breast as a second stage of the same procedure. Biopsy specimens should be carefully studied, and too many mistakes have been made when surgery was done on the basis of a hasty pathology report made while the patient was still on the operating table. Evaluation of a frozen section is likely to be less accurate than a thorough study that takes a couple of days.

When you receive the biopsy report and find that cancer has been diagnosed, ask your doctor to get a second opinion on the slides from a different pathologist. False reports are not uncommon and, if you are diagnosed as having cancer, it is folly not to make sure that the pathologist is right. If the diagnosis is confirmed by a second pathologist, it is time to discuss with your surgeon the treatment alternatives that are available.

If your surgeon is conscientious and compassionate, and not so dedicated to radical surgery that he will consider nothing else, he will gladly discuss the options that are open to you and their relative merits and demerits in your individual case. At that point, the choice among the potential risks and benefits should be yours to make.

I must warn you, however, to be prepared for the possibility of strong resistance and cavalier treatment from the surgeon when he discovers that you are not going to submit, uninformed and passive, to his advice. You may have encountered someone who believes he is God. Don't be intimidated into signing a release for surgery. Demand a signed agreement that the surgeon will not go beyond the biopsy that you have agreed to let him perform. Don't authorize any form of treatment without a thorough discussion of the alternatives. Get a second opinion, and get a new doctor if it appears that your surgeon is one who always insists on a radical mastectomy because he doesn't like to do anything else.

11

"It's Safer Than Pregnancy."

The Pill was approved for sale by the FDA in 1960, after five years of research funded by the birth control advocate Margaret Sanger and the drug manufacturer G. D. Searle. Millions of women, delighted to obtain a convenient, effective means of birth control, eagerly began using the drug. Because it was given to them by their doctors and had been approved by the federal pharmaceutical watchdogs, they assumed that it could be taken without risk. They couldn't have been more wrong.

FDA approval of the Pill was based on careless, inadequate studies that established its effectiveness but offered no valid scientific proof that it was safe for human use. One of the studies involved 132 Puerto Rican women who took the Pill for a year or more. *Five of them died during the study, and no effort was even made to find out why!* On the basis of that kind of "scientific evidence" the FDA approved a drug that ultimately would endanger 50 million women all over the world.

With the encouragement of their physicians, women have

been swallowing the Pill for twenty years. To this day, no one has been able to offer conclusive evidence that it is safe for human use. Doctors continue to prescribe oral contraceptives despite repeated instances of adverse effects that they see in their patients and an abundance of evidence in the scientific journals that they are responsible for a host of ills and countless deaths.

Not long after birth control pills were introduced, doctors began observing a wide range of dangerous and even deadly effects from the conjugated estrogens that they contain. Over the next two decades, more than 100 studies linked use of the drug to more than fifty adverse effects. The FDA responded by demanding innocuous warning labels about some of them, but failed to protect women by halting distribution of the Pill.

Typically, the drug manufacturers responded to each of the studies with the double negative defense that they always employ: *There is no conclusive scientific evidence that oral contraceptives are not safe for human use.* How many bodies must be laid at their door before the drug manufacturers abandon this cynical defense?

As a doctor, I find the original FDA decision to permit sale of the Pill without extensive testing an incomprehensible one. The adverse effects of the Pill were predictable, and the short-term damage would have been detected had its sponsors been as interested in checking its safety as they were in demonstrating that it worked.

Problems with oral contraceptives were predictable because of the way they affect the body. Don't expect to hear this from your doctor, because the Pill wouldn't have many takers if women were told that it alters hormonal balance to create a physiological dysfunction. The desired result is to interfere with a natural process—ovulation—by causing the body to malfunction. Thus, the Pill literally makes every woman who takes it sick. For some women, the immediate symptoms are mild and scarcely noticeable; for others, they are severe. But all of those who take it are exposed to potentially deadly risks.

Interfering with the functions of the reproductive system is bad enough, but the Pill's effects do not stop there. The estrogens affect every cell, every organ in the body. The undesired effects on other organs also vary from one user to another, but they include acute discomfort, serious disease, and even untimely death. Because most of the Pill's insidious effects are not immediately apparent, women take it without suspicion that it is hurting them. After all, the damage may not appear for twenty or more years.

Over the last two decades I have read scores of scientific studies revealing the diseases and mortality rates suffered by users of the Pill. These women have been shown to have a higher incidence of cancer of the cervix, uterus, breast, and liver. The Pill has also been linked to heart attacks, strokes, diabetes, gall bladder disease, pulmonary embolism, hypertension, and mental depression. Some women who take the Pill as a means of family planning discover to their dismay that it has made them permanently sterile when they try to have a child. To these major effects can be added a score or more of lesser symptoms, ranging from vaginal infections and breast enlargement to the loss of hair on the scalp and the growth of hair on the face.

If doctors kept abreast of the medical literature and acted on the basis of what they read, they should long ago have turned their backs on the Pill. There is no rational excuse for risking damage or death for their patients when safe and equally reliable options are available. Yet, despite the catalog of horrors associated with oral contraceptives, the FDA continues to approve them for human use. Drug manufacturers continue to fatten their purses by making and selling them. Doctors continue to prescribe them for millions of American women, while the population controllers peddle them to unsuspecting women all over the world.

It is hard for me to believe that this travesty has been allowed to continue for twenty years!

It may be instructive to you, as it was to me, to compare the way the FDA coddles the drug manufacturers with the way they responded in 1980 when the Rely tampon was linked to toxic shock syndrome. Although only two inconclusive studies suggested that the Rely tampon was the culprit, and although only forty deaths had been reported from toxic shock syndrome during the previous five years, the FDA promptly bombarded the press with vigorous warnings about the product.

An official of the FDA boasted to the *Wall Street Journal* that his agency had deliberately used the media to drive the product off the market. "We wanted to saturate the market with information on Rely," he said. "We deliberately delayed issuing press releases to maximize media impact. There was quite a concerted and deliberate effort to keep a steady flow of information before the public."

I'd like to hear him explain why the FDA hasn't been equally vigorous in protecting American women from far more dangerous products, such as birth control pills and intrauterine devices (IUDs), which have been on the market for twenty years!

The participants in the sinister Pill conspiracy continue to justify their behavior by asserting that the end—population control—justifies the means. Doctors, who are most culpable because it lies in their power to stop prescribing the Pill, defend using it in the face of known risks because, they say, it is safer than pregnancy. Even if that were true, that argument would make no sense. Other safe, equally reliable forms of contraception are available to prevent pregnancy. More directly to the point, however, is the fact that the mortality rate from the Pill—when all of its fatal effects are combined—is infinitely greater than the risk of death from pregnancy. One study revealed a death rate twenty times that of pregnancy from Pill-related vascular diseases alone.

I can recall a time when the modal age range of breast cancer victims was forty-five to fifty-five years. Doctors rarely, if ever, saw young women with the disease. The modal age range has moved down into the thirty-year bracket since women began taking the Pill. Those who studied one group of 450 women were shocked to find fifteen cases of breast cancer among women between the ages of fifteen and twenty-nine. *All fifteen of these young women were taking the Pill.*

To put the hazards of oral contraceptives in perspective, let me remind you that nonprofit health agencies have been formed to combat diseases that cause fewer deaths than the Pill. However, I haven't seen any of my colleagues holding tag days for the victims of oral contraceptives that they prescribe. It is a rare doctor who tells his patients that the drug might kill them, and some even deny their patients the right to make a less risky choice. It makes me angry, sick at heart, and ashamed of my profession when I receive letters such as this from female readers:

About nine years ago, when reports began surfacing about the link between the Pill and cancer and blood clots, I went to my gynecologist to ask to be fitted for a diaphragm. After the birth of my first child, this doctor had put me on the contraceptive pill (although I had not asked for it), assuring me that it would not only act as a birth control device, but would also protect me against cancer.

After being positioned and draped by the nurse, I heard the doctor coming in, gaily humming, "Well, hello, Mrs. Robinson." When he discovered I wanted to be taken off the Pill, he became angry and said he would not fit me for a diaphragm. He told me if I went off the Pill I was on my own. He advised me to "go down to the drug store, get some foam and take your chances."

A friend of mine who is a nurse suffered considerable water retention while she was on the Pill, so her gynecologist gave her a diuretic. After a while, the combination of the contraceptive pill and the diuretic began to produce symptoms of diabetes. The doctor then wanted to prescribe a third medication to control the diabetes. When my friend refused, the doctor suggested a hysterectomy as an alternative.

I think many gynecologists do not like women. If a woman is young, dumb and/or sexy, the gynecologist may find her tolerable, but he considers the rest of us to be less than human.

Periodically, when the mounting evidence of the Pill's dangers begins making women wary of its use, new studies are trotted out and widely publicized to dispel their doubts. They do their dirty work and then fade into oblivion when their biases are exposed. One of the classics was a study publicized by Planned Parenthood-World Population. It was said to prove that Pill users didn't suffer catastrophic effects. Subsequently, it was revealed that the design of the study included only long-time users of the Pill *and excluded the victims who were already dead.*

In late 1980, two decades after the introduction of oral contraceptives, I picked up my newspaper one morning and was greeted by a bold headline that read: "Risks from Birth Control Pill Negligible, Study Says." The article was based on a ten-year study done at the Kaiser-Permanente Medical Center at Walnut Creek, California. It left the impression that oral contraceptives had at last been proven to be safe.

A few phone calls revealed that the summary of the study, funded by the National Institute of Child Health and Human Development, had been rushed to the media without waiting for publication of the complete report. This assured that the publicity would achieve its objective, because millions of women would be reassured about the Pill before knowledgeable scientists were able to study the report and challenge the results.

When I managed to get a copy of the summary, it was immediately apparent that the reassurances it provided were all in the headlines, not in the report. The summary contained so many qualifications and disclaimers that it proved nothing at all.

First of all, the findings were applicable only to young, adult, healthy, white, middle-class American women who lived in California and were enrolled in the same prepaid health care plan. They did not apply to those who are in high-risk groups because they smoke, had early sexual experiences or multiple sex partners, or may get cancer because they spend too much time in the sun.

Apparently, assuming that Kaiser-Permanente is practicing conscientious medicine, the study also did not apply to women who had previously been warned not to take the Pill because they were significantly overweight or severely depressed, because they were suffering from high blood pressure or migraine headaches, or because they were pregnant or breast-feeding. The "reassuring" findings are also inapplicable to women with varicose veins or a history of blood clotting disorders, liver abnormalities, sickle cell anemia, glaucoma, large fibroid tumors, or diabetes, or a family history of same.

The authors also noted that their study did not compare the risks of oral contraceptives with those of other forms of birth control, or with the risks of pregnancy, *and did not evaluate the effects of Pill use on subsequent fertility.* Finally, the study warned that because the long-range effects of the Pill are not known, "The final word on oral contraceptives is not yet in."

Even if I try to be charitable, I can't imagine what purpose—other than misleading women about the safety of the Pill—the report served. Certainly, it did not merit the blanket assertion in the headline that risks to women from the Pill are negligible.

The lack of concern of doctors for the health and lives of their patients has also been evident where IUDs are concerned. Since the late 1960s, millions of American women have been supplied with these dangerous devices by their physicians. Some of them simply wanted to delay starting their families, and others who already had the children they wanted were looking for a convenient, reliable method of birth control. When they allowed their doctors to insert the devices, few of them realized that the IUD could make them permanently sterile, perforate the uterus and migrate into the abdominal cavity, or cause pelvic inflammatory disease (PID). In 1974, the FDA released figures that linked thirty-nine deaths to IUDs. Since 1970 more than a million women have suffered acute pelvic infections attributable to the devices. It is estimated that 20 percent of them—as many as 250,000 women—have been or will be rendered sterile by IUD-induced PID.

No one is precisely certain how an IUD acts to prevent pregnancy, but it is believed that the presence of the device in the uterus causes an inflammation of the uterine lining that is hostile to the implantation of a fertilized egg. When an egg is deposited in the uterus by the fallopian tube, it is expelled. Thus, the IUD is not really a contraceptive barrier to the fertilization of the egg. Instead, it causes an abortion when conception occurs.

The insertion of foreign objects into the uterus as a means of birth control dates back at least two thousand years. Until the early 1960s, when they were co-opted by the population control proponents, American doctors refused to use them because they caused infections, peritonitis, and death. Only twenty years ago the use of IUDs was considered a form of malpractice, and warnings against their use were given to students in medical schools.

As the population control movement gained strength in the United States, attention was again focused on the IUD. It was attractive because it could be inserted into poor, uneducated women who were not strongly motivated to stop having kids. Once it was inserted, the family planners no longer had to worry about whether the women would take the trouble to use a diaphragm or remember to take the Pill. A device like that was too tempting to pass up, despite the risks of infertility and death. (I'm tempted to note that sterility and death are remarkably effective means of preventing pregnancy, too.)

In 1962, the Population Council held an international conference to promote the IUD, and the devices came into their own. Dr. J. Robert Willson, of the University of Michigan School of Medicine, apparently reflected the view of the doctors who attended when he said:

> If we look at this from an overall, long-range view—these are things I have never said out loud before, and I don't know how it is going to sound—*perhaps the individual patient is expendable in the general scheme of things,* particularly if the infection she acquires is sterilizing but not lethal. (Italics added.)

I can understand why Dr. Willson was concerned about how that argument would sound. If his audience had been women instead of doctors, they would have been outraged. What is left of the tattered fabric of medical ethics if doctors have decided that their individual patients are "expendable" in the pursuit of social goals?

I'm sure that the doctors who attended the conference weren't visualizing their affluent white patients when they sanctioned use of the IUD. The "expendables" were the poverty-stricken, uneducated racial minorities in the United States and women in Africa, Asia, and the underdeveloped nations of the world. Inevitably, however, this discriminatory distinction was blurred. American women of all races and all classes became the guinea pigs on whom IUDs were tested, *and they still are.*

This massive experiment on American women soon revealed a disastrous fact. In their haste to stem the tide of dark-skinned babies, all of the conspirators failed to consider a new hazard that the seven most widely used IUDs had in common. Each of them had a string attached that descended from the uterus into the vagina. This innovation—not present in earlier German-made IUDS—was designed to enable women to determine whether their IUD was in place and to make the device easier to remove.

At the outset doctors overlooked the fact that the strings provided an inviting path for bacteria to travel from the vagina into the uterus—and when this became known, they chose to ignore it. Because the lining of the uterus was irritated by the IUD, the bacteria found a hospitable environment in which to produce pelvic inflammatory disease. The infection could then spread to the ovaries and the fallopian tubes, often scarring the latter so that conception could never occur.

The doctors who inserted IUDs in their patients knew, although their patients probably didn't, that the devices were not subject to federal supervision or control. The manufacturers were free to market them with little or no previous testing. Doctors exploited their patients to learn, from the complications that these women suffered, whether or not IUDs were safe.

I find it unforgivable that doctors are still inflicting IUDs on their patients when, after twenty years, there is still no precise, reliable information about the adverse effects of the IUD. No one knows what the mortality rate is, although death certainly is one of the IUD's effects. No one knows the extent of the long-range side effects from the IUD. No one knows the incidence of permanent sterility from its use or the number of ectopic pregnancies it causes. No one knows the incidence of cancer of the cervix resulting from its use. No one even knows for sure what the upper limits are of the incidence of PID.

One device, the Dalkon Shield, was actually placed on the market and advertised as exceptionally safe on the basis of altered test results. The manufacturer continued to sell it even after its own researchers advised management that it had a uniquely dangerous element. The shield used a multifilament string that drew bacteria into the uterus because it acted as a wick.

About 2½ million Dalkon Shields were sold in the United States between January 1971 and June 1974, when the manufacturer, A. H. Robins Co., removed the product from the market. Seventeen deaths have been associated with use of the shield, and by the end of 1979, the company's insurer had settled some 2,400 claims arising from adverse effects from this IUD. Only a few claims were allowed to go to court, and in one of those a thirty-year-old Denver woman was awarded $6.8 million. She had become pregnant while wearing the shield, spontaneously aborted, required a total hysterectomy, and then suffered migraine headaches and severe depression.

My advice to any woman whose doctor suggests that she use an intrauterine device is that she ask him how expendable he considers *her*.

I fully appreciate that safe and reliable forms of contraception, such as the diaphragm and the Billings method, may be a nuisance and less appealing than the IUD and the Pill. Still, I am sure that women, if given the facts, would agree that inconvenience is a small price to pay for survival and continued health.

As you undoubtedly know, Planned Parenthood is one of the population control agencies that has promoted the IUD and the

Pill with a hard-sell approach. Before you consider using either of these methods, you should know how they are regarded by the Planned Parenthood women who peddle them to others.

A survey done among 800 of Planned Parenthood's female staff members revealed a striking aversion to the Pill. Only 8.8 percent of these women take contraceptive pills, but 70 percent of their clients do. Thirty-eight percent of the Planned Parenthood workers choose to use the diaphragm, but only 9 percent of their clients do.

The doctor who conducted the study had a simple explanation for these disparities: The Planned Parenthood workers shied away from the Pill because they were exposed every day to clients who suffered from its harmful effects. However, the women they were counseling were willing to take it because they were unaware of the harm the Pill could cause!

12

"Now Look, Mother, You've Got to Watch Your Weight."

If doctors fail to keep women from becoming pregnant, they will do their utmost to make the experience as unpleasant as possible. They do it by persuading prospective mothers that a normal physiological process is really a life-threatening nine-month disease.

Women experiencing their first pregnancy are sent to prenatal classes, presumably to be informed and reassured, but actually to be softened up for all of the needless intervention that their obstetricians have in store for them. Doctors know they can't afford to allow their patients to perceive childbirth as the normal, typically uncomplicated process that it really is. If they did, most women wouldn't need obstetricians. What many women don't realize is that more often than not, it is the unnecessary intervention of doctors that causes most of the complications that they are taught to fear.

As a pediatrician, I am revolted by the consequences of this dangerous intervention that I see in the babies entrusted to my

130

care. The damage that is done to them begins right after the good news comes back from the rabbit, when the mother-to-be is admonished to watch her weight and told to limit the gain to a specific number of pounds. That number is inversely proportional to the stupidity of the doctor who is making the rules.

Half a century or so ago, when people still realized that grandmothers were usually smarter than doctors, pregnant women heeded the advice that they were "eating for two." Today, many obstetricians won't let their patients eat enough for one. For many years, doctors tried to limit weight gain during pregnancy to ten or fifteen pounds. Some idiots still do. More recently, though, most doctors have become more generous and raised the ante to twenty or twenty-five pounds, which is less dangerous but still wrong.

It's wrong because the health of mother and baby is not determined by the amount of weight the mother gains, but by the quality of the food she consumes. Every pregnant woman should be on a diet that includes sufficient calories, protein, vitamins, and minerals. She should take special care to get an adequate supply of calcium and iron—not from pills, but from the foods she eats. An intake of two quarts of fluid a day is desirable and necessary to cope with expanding blood volume. Furthermore, whatever your doctor may tell you, a healthy woman experiencing a normal pregnancy has no need to restrict salt. Salt is also needed to maintain the blood volume necessary to nourish both mother and child.

During my years of pediatric practice I've been visited by an endless stream of mothers and babies who display the consequences of excessive weight control and poor nutrition. That's why I was not surprised in 1975 when a federal agency reported that about one of every three pregnant American women suffers from malnutrition—nearly a million women a year, in all. Some of these women are malnourished because of poverty, of course. An inordinate number, however, are undernourished not because they can't afford to eat, but because their doctors won't let them eat well.

Physicians are indoctrinated in medical school to demand

that their patients control their weight during pregnancy. Meanwhile, they are taught little or nothing about a pregnant woman's nutritional needs. I don't know of a medical school in the country that requires its students to learn anything at all about nutrition. That's just another evidence of Modern Medicine's preoccupation with intervention rather than prevention in the practice of its art. Veterinarians know more about diets for pregnant animals than doctors know about the nutritional needs of the pregnant women in their care.

The disastrous consequence of this nutritional ignorance, combined with compulsive intervention, is a Pandora's box of needless complications for mother and child. Despite the common belief among doctors that it is more difficult to deliver a baby whose mother is overweight, the reverse is actually true. Numerous studies have shown that when mothers are malnourished the uterus may not function properly and labor is prolonged or even stops. Having created the problem with his arbitrary weight control standards, the obstetrician then creates more problems by inducing labor. If that fails, he hits the jackpot and delivers the baby by Caesarean section. This is a pattern that I have observed repeatedly throughout the practice of Modern Medicine. By encouraging the mother to restrict her weight, the doctor creates the conditions that make it necessary for him to intervene. Studies have shown that complications are experienced by half the mothers with low birth-weight babies, but they appear in only 10 percent of mothers who have babies of normal weight.

For years doctors believed, and many still do, that overweight mothers were more likely to develop toxemia—one of pregnancy's most dangerous and sometimes fatal complications. Yet, for half a century, evidence has been accumulating that maternal nutrition—not weight gain—is the cause. The absence of the proper nutritional elements in the mother's diet causes the liver to malfunction, and the body's responses produce the symptoms that are associated with toxemia. Once again, the doctor's own ignorance of nutrition is the cause of the disease.

Many doctors also display an utter lack of understanding of

the swelling due to water retention that occurs in at least 80 percent of women at some time during pregnancy. With limited exceptions, this is a normal and healthy condition because the stored fluid that causes the edema helps provide an adequate supply to support the increased blood volume that mother and baby need. Many doctors don't know this, and because they have been taught to regard swelling as an indication of toxemia, they seize on it as another excuse to intervene.

They have had the usual encouragement from the drug manufacturers, of course, who always welcome another non-disease. Drugs promoted for the treatment of maternal edema are featured in page after page of four-color medical journal ads. Doctors, who ought to know better, prescribe them to eliminate the very fluids that the mother and the fetus need. It has been reported that more than 90 percent of doctors caring for pregnant women have prescribed diuretics and that some 2 million pregnant women are treated with them every year.

In the event that an obstetrician tries to give you diuretics, you should be aware that the results can be catastrophic in two respects. First, the death rate of infants born to mothers without edema has been shown to be nearly 50 percent higher than among those who retain an extra supply of fluid. Second, for some rather complex reasons, if the mother really has toxemia and is treated with diuretics, the drug can kill her by lowering her blood pressure and pushing her into hypovolemic shock. That occurs simply because she does not have an adequate blood supply to support normal bodily functions.

As a pediatrician, I am most troubled about what a deliberately malnourished mother does to her child. If her obstetrician holds her to an arbitrary maximum weight, she is likely to be pushing the upper limits during the final two months of pregnancy. This compels her to reduce food intake during precisely the period of greatest weight gain for her unborn child—just to keep her doctor happy. She literally starves her baby, endangering its health and life, as well as her own. To make matters worse, the baby is denied adequate nutrition during the final crucial period in the development of its brain.

A diet of high-quality foods is the best insurance a mother can have against delivering a low-birth-weight child. A well-nourished woman who gains thirty or even forty pounds will have a better chance of delivering a healthy eight-pound baby. A mother who starves herself in order to satisfy her obstetrician's criminally rigid standards of weight gain is likely to deliver a baby of less than five pounds.

The consequences suffered by low-birth-weight babies are manifold. I have seen them in my own practice, day after day, and the statistics tell me as much or more. The chances that an underweight baby will die during the first twenty-eight days after delivery are thirty times those of babies born at normal weight. Mental retardation is found in half of the low-birth-weight babies, and they also have three times the incidence of epilepsy, cerebral palsy, and learning and behavioral problems as do babies of normal weight.

There isn't much you can do to educate your doctor about nutrition. However, if you can't find one who values it, you can educate yourself. A good way to start is to read the book *What Every Pregnant Woman Should Know,* by Gail and Tom Brewer. Dr. Tom Brewer is president of the Society for the Protection of the Unborn Through Nutrition (SPUN). I'm so concerned about the nutritional damage I see in the infants I treat that I agreed to become vice-president of the group.

What you learn probably won't help you convert your obstetrician. (After all, "Where did *you* go to medical school?") It will help you to have a healthy baby, even if your doctor is giving you lousy medical advice.

13

"Don't Tell Me You Want to Be a Martyr!"

Doctors have contorted every aspect of pregnancy into a profitable and often dangerous opportunity to intervene. If you become pregnant and want the experience to be a happy and natural one, be prepared to do battle with your obstetrician— every step of the way. Make it clear from the outset that you intend to retain control over your own destiny and that of your child.

Your first opportunity to resist needless and potentially hazardous intervention may come if you develop the nausea and vomiting that are associated with "morning sickness." About half of the women who become pregnant experience it to some degree, as women have for thousands of years. The symptoms usually disappear by the end of the fourth month of pregnancy, and until then they can be minimized by following a proper diet.

When I was in medical school, doctors tried to make something pathological out of morning sickness by giving it a medical name. They called it hyperemesis gravidarum, which means excessive vomiting because of pregnancy, but the name didn't stick. Until about a quarter of a century ago, doctors were frustrated because women were treating themselves with herbal remedies and no drug was available that would enable them to intervene. As might be expected, the profit potential of a treatment for morning sickness wasn't lost on the drug manufacturers, either. One of them came up with the product that was the answer to the obstetricians' prayers.

The new drug first surfaced in October 1954, in a memo sent to the president of the Richardson-Merrell pharmaceutical firm by a member of his research staff. It described a new compound that could be promoted for use in treating nausea and vomiting in pregnant women.

> Between three million and four million pregnancies occur annually in the United States and will continue within that range for some time to come, [the researcher wrote]. About half the pregnant women I used to see in the prenatal clinic, when I was an obstetrical resident, complained of enough nausea and vomiting *to justify writing a prescription for some safe and probably effective medication.* (Italics added.)

The profit potential of an exclusive new drug that might be sold to 4 million women a year struck a responsive chord in the Richardson-Merrell pursestrings. In 1957 the company applied for, and in just twenty-eight days received, FDA approval to market a product named Bendectin for the treatment of nausea and vomiting in early pregnancy.

Bendectin is the only drug marketed in the United States for specific use by women during the first trimester of pregnancy. It is one too many, because this is the critical period during which most of the development of the limbs and organs of the fetus occurs. Yet the new drug was greeted enthusiastically by doctors, who were overjoyed to have "a probably effective medication" that they could prescribe for morning sickness.

Bendectin, marketed under this and other names, was soon

being sold in thirty-one countries. It has been used by about 30 million women since it was placed on the market in 1957. It fulfilled the expectations of its manufacturer, because 1.5 million women take it every year. Less certain is whether it fulfilled the expectations of the women who took it, because there are serious questions about whether it really works.

It is important for you to know that Richardson-Merrell has a history that does not inspire confidence. In 1958, two years after Bendectin was introduced, the company obtained from the German drug firm Chemie Grunenthal the United States rights to market Thalidomide. In late 1960, although Thalidomide had not been approved by the FDA for sale in the United States, Richardson-Merrell began distributing samples of the drug to American doctors for experimental use with their patients. *The distribution to doctors in this country continued even after the drug was withdrawn in Germany because it was believed to cause horrible birth defects.*

Fortunately for American women *and* for Richardson-Merrell, a determined woman scientist at the FDA blocked approval of the drug for marketing in the United States. Although some of the women who had been given the sample pills by their doctors gave birth to deformed children, the FDA's caution spared other thousands from its terrible effects.

Richardson-Merrell was also the developer of MER 29, a drug developed to control the body's metabolism of cholesterol and marketed for the treatment of arteriosclerosis. Soon after it was introduced, doctors who prescribed the drug began reporting side effects that included nausea, loss of hair, a severe skin ailment called ichthyosis, and cataracts of the eye. Richardson-Merrell failed to reveal the side effects that were reported to it and continued to market the drug.

The hazards of MER 29 came to light two years later, after the FDA learned that a Merrell laboratory technician had been ordered to falsify the results of animal tests on MER 29. An FDA investigation revealed that MER 29 caused cataracts and ichthyosis. Criminal indictments were brought against the company and three of its executives. They pleaded "no contest," and the company received the maximum fine—$80,000—and the executives were placed on probation for six months.

This unsavory track record makes me look with considerable skepticism at the defenses that Richardson-Merrell is now advancing for Bendectin. There are strong indications that history is repeating itself. The research that was presented to the FDA to secure approval of Bendectin was totally inadequate. Although the drug was intended specifically for use by pregnant women, no research was done to determine whether it might cause defects in the unborn child.

Only after the Thalidomide scandal broke was such testing done. All but two of the rabbits used in the first test died because of a sudden drop in temperature in the lab, and there were no abnormalities reported in the offspring of those that survived. A second test was performed and the company reported abnormalities in only two of the forty-eight kits that were born—not enough to conclude that the drug caused birth defects. Not until seventeen years later, when the company records were brought to light in court, did women learn that the company had inaccurately reported the Bendectin test results. A reexamination of the test data revealed that abnormalities had appeared in one of every eight rabbit kits born during the tests, not one in twenty-four!

The published research on Bendectin strongly suggests that the drug may cause birth defects. Dr. Jose Cardero, at the Center for Disease Control in Atlanta, reviewed 250,000 births and associated Bendectin with limb reduction defects—such as missing hands and feet—and a devastating abnormality in which the brain is formed outside the skull. Another study suggested that nearly five birth defects could be expected among the children of each 1,000 mothers who took Bendectin during the first trimester of pregnancy.

Thalidomide produced shocking birth defects in 20 percent of the children of mothers who took it. The observed incidence of birth defects in the children of Bendectin users is considereably lower, but over the long term that may be the most sinister characteristic of all. It will make it more difficult to develop the conclusive evidence that is needed to compel the FDA to halt its sale.

At this writing, Richarson-Merrell still maintains that Bendectin is safe, and the FDA continues to permit its sale. By some curious reasoning process, the company even claimed vindication for its product when a Florida jury awarded damages to a Bendectin user who gave birth to a deformed child.

The birth of a defective baby is a tragedy for all those involved, and one with secondary consequences that are also of great concern. The parents of a defective child are often inclined to blame themselves or each other, believing that some genetic aberration must be the cause. The psychological consequences for the mother can be extreme and—not knowing that drugs rather than genetics were responsible—she may decide never to have another child.

Teratogenesis, the medical term used to describe drug-induced birth defects, is an ugly word. It derives from the Latin word *terato,* meaning monster, and its literal meaning is "the creation of monsters." Whether Bendectin is a teratogen has not been established conclusively, nor has anyone established conclusively that it is not. However, the files of the manufacturer and the FDA contain many reports of deformed infants born to mothers after its use.

There is ample evidence that some drugs taken by the mother during the early months of pregnancy will cross the placental barrier and damage the fetus. How many others will do so is unknown, but the hazards are sufficiently grave that no doctor should prescribe *any* drugs for pregnant women unless he has a life-saving reason to do so. I believe that any doctor who prescribes a possible teratogen for relief of a minor symptom like nausea is one whom every prudent woman should avoid.

If your doctor tries to give you Bendectin, ask yourself whether relief from your nausea is important enough to risk depriving your baby of its hands or feet. After you have told him what he can do with the drug, start worrying about what a doctor who prescribes a suspected teratogen for a pregnant patient will try to do to you next.

14

"Do You Want Your Baby to Die?"

An expectant mother should thank Providence for her good fortune if she has her baby in a taxicab on the way to the hospital. The cab driver may not be much help, but at least he will spare her from all of the purposeless, perilous, and unpleasant intervention her obstetrician had planned to inflict on her. If the new mother has her wits about her she'll ask the driver to wait, have the cord cut in the hospital emergency room, and then get back in the cab and take her baby home.

Ideally, she shouldn't have been in the cab in the first place, because the safest place for a healthy mother to have her baby is not in a hospital, but at home. Unfortunately, it isn't easy for her to make that choice, because most doctors won't attend a birth if the mother refuses to go to the hospital. Obstetricians don't lose much business by being so arbitrary because most pregnant women don't even ask to have their babies at home. They're afraid to, because their obstetrician has so convincingly described the perils of natural, home birth, that they reluctantly accept the "protection" of the hospital. They dread going there but conclude they must do so to assure the health and safety of their unborn child.

If the prospective mother is insistent on home birth, she can expect her doctor to terminate the conversation by drawing himself up to full height and asking her sternly, "Do you want your baby to die?" There are two ways to answer that question. One is to reply, "No, that's why I want to have it at home." An even better response is "Good-bye!"

I've observed that doctors are as skilled as carnival pitchmen—and just as deceptive—when it comes to touting the "marvels of medical technology" that are at their disposal in the hospital "in case something goes wrong." Equally vivid are their self-serving warnings about the hazards of having your baby at home. Words seem to fail them, though, when it comes to confessing the truth about the medical booby traps that await you within the hospital walls.

Your doctor won't tell you, so I will: your own bedroom is safer than the hospital delivery room, and the hospital nursery is infinitely more threatening to your baby than a crib next to your bed. I tell all healthy women, including my own daughters, that they should refuse to have their babies in the hospital precisely *because* of the potentially dangerous technological wizardry that is available to their doctor there.

I have always told my patients that they should avoid hospitals as they would avoid war. Do your utmost to stay out of them and, if you find yourself in one, do everything possible to get out as soon as you can. After working in hospitals for most of my life, I can assure you that they are the dirtiest and most deadly places in town.

That may not square with your perception of all those glistening corridors and sparkling white sheets. I'll grant that most hospitals *look* awesomely antiseptic, but if you examined them with a microscope you'd know that they are not. They are actually so germ-laden that 5 percent of all hospital patients contract new infections that they didn't have when they arrived. As a result, they are stuck there for an average of seven extra days.

In a single year, 1.5 million patients were victims of hospital-acquired infections and about 15,000 of them died. Understandably, Modern Medicine is so fearful that you'll discover its role in spreading disease that medical texts caution doctors not to allow the phrase *hospital-acquired infections* to pass their lips. They're told to conceal the truth from their patients by using the term *nosocomial infections* instead. That will keep all of their patients in the dark except the ones who speak Greek. Of course, whatever you call the fatal infections, the patients who contract them are still just as dead.

One study of hospital costs claims that the money devoted to reducing the risks of infection is only a tenth of what is needed. I can't help wondering if that is because the average infection produces the revenue from seven extra patient-days. Many of the infections could be prevented by better training and supervision, but there isn't much evidence that those in charge really care.

Germs are transmitted from one patient to another by careless doctors and nurses who don't scrub often or well enough, and carry bacteria from one patient to another on their hands. For obvious reasons, hospitals are vacation spas for potentially lethal bacteria, and you'll find them everywhere you turn. They are on the wheelchairs and on the gurneys that are used to convey live patients to surgery and dead patients from surgery to the morgue. They are in the pillows and the mattresses, camouflaged but not constrained by the white pillowcases and sheets. They are distributed from one room to another by the mops and the dust cloths, and clouds of germs are blown all over the building through the heating and air conditioning ducts.

Your hospital bill will be filled with charges for disposable everything, which is justified as a means of making sure that the items used on you are sterile and clean. Yet, that stethoscope that dangles around the doctor's neck is pressed against the bare flesh of patient after patient without being sterilized in between. The fabric of the blood pressure cuff is a motel for all of the bacteria that other patients have carried through the hospital doors.

And then there's the food. I've seen outbreaks of infectious hepatitis transmitted from kitchen workers to patients who unwittingly munched the virus along with their meals. If you are unlucky enough to encounter a contaminated batch of intravenous fluid, you are not even safe when they feed you through your veins. In fact, you can't be sure that any supposedly sterile bottle of anything is really pure. One curious health official tested the bottles of saline solution that were kept on bedside tables for use in cleansing wounds. He found potentially pathogenic bacteria in nearly one bottle out of four.

All of these germs are hazards to the mother, of course. They are even more threatening to the newborn babies, whose immune systems are not yet fully developed. Low-birth-weight babies are at particular risk. A study conducted in a Utah intensive care unit found hospital-acquired infections in 24.6 percent of the babies, compared with 7.3 percent of the patients in the hospital overall. The diseases transmitted to the babies were also more serious than those found in the adult patients in other areas of the hospital. The infections were spread by contact with the nursing staff and with nursery equipment, and through invasive procedures such as antibiotic shots. A similar twenty-one-week study done at the University of Iowa hospital intensive care nursery found that 21 percent of the babies acquired infections while they were there.

Premature babies in hospital nurseries may also become the victims of the technology that is supposed to keep them well. A condition called retrolental fibroplasia, which results in partial or total blindness, has been caused by administering excessive concentrations of oxygen to premature babies in airtight incubators. Other babies have suffered first-degree burns from the radiant warmers in which they were placed.

I am also concerned that the obligatory ritual of placing silver nitrate in the eyes of the newborn—theoretically to guard against gonorrheal infection—may be responsible for the higher incidence of astigmatism and myopia in the United States than in countries that don't perform this ridiculous rite. It's a useless procedure, and there is no scientific basis to believe that it's safe, yet in many states it is required by law. I tell my students to comply with the law but to do it by squirting the chemical in the general direction of the baby from ten feet away.

The mandatory use of silver nitrate in the eyes of the newborn is one of the most revealing examples of Modern Medicine's attitude toward women. One of the things I was taught in medical school was how to take a patient's history. If I asked a patient whether she had ever had high blood pressure and she said, "No," I was to write down, "No." If I asked her whether she had ever had a venereal disease and she said, "No," I was to write down, "Patient denies venereal disease."

Just as some religions have their original sin, medicine has its original disease. When a woman is pregnant, doctors proceed on the assumption she has gonorrhea. They don't look for it in the mother. Instead, they simply assume that she is infected and when the baby is born they put silver nitrate drops in its eyes. That doesn't really do any good because if the baby does develop gonorrheal ophthalmia, it still has to be treated with penicillin or another powerful antibiotic.

Unfortunately for the baby, silver nitrate can do harm. Its side effects include blocked tear ducts during the first six months of life and, more important, a chemical conjunctivitis that prevents the newborn baby from seeing. That doesn't bother doctors because they believe that babies can't see for the first couple of days, anyway. The reason they believe that is that the newborn babies they observe have all had silver nitrate put into their eyes. I also believed they couldn't see until my granddaughter was born in my house and didn't receive silver nitrate. She looked at me and I could tell that she was seeing me.

If your baby escapes the infections and other threats rampant in the nursery, there is still the risk that it will simply disappear. Cases of kidnapping from hospital nurseries are reported every year. They are still looking for a baby kidnapped from the newborn nursery of Michael Reese Hospital in Chicago many years ago. The child is now almost old enough to begin looking for its mother.

Even more likely is the possibility that a mix-up in the nursery will send you home with the wrong baby. Occasionally these errors result in lawsuits, but they usually do not. That's simply because mothers see so little of their babies while they are in the hospital that they would be hard put to know or to prove whether or not they got the right one.

Mothers and babies alike are also endangered by the carelessness and inefficiency that can be found in even the best hospitals in the land. You always have to worry that the nurse might give you the wrong pill or an injection meant for somebody else. A study in one 300-bed hospital showed that the nurses gave a patient the wrong medication once in every seven times they had the chance. The average patient gets twelve different drugs during a hospital stay, so those are frightening odds. Some patients die because they are given the wrong medication. One of the most shocking cases I have seen recently was that of the mother of seven children who died because a big city hospital pharmacy gave her medicine intended for somebody else.

Patients have died in hospitals because the lines that carried oxygen and those that transported nitrous oxide were accidentally reversed. Others have suffered from hemorrhage because nurses mistakenly attached oxygen tanks to stomach tubes; the surgical stitches ripped out when the patient's stomach blew up like a balloon. Still other patients have succumbed to intravenous feeding with contaminated fluids or transfusions of the wrong type of blood.

If nothing else in the hospital kills you, there is always the possibility that you will starve to death. It is not so much that the food is nutritionally inadequate; it is just that most of it tastes so bad that the patients refuse to eat it, and there is no one around who will make sure they do. Consequently, malnutrition is a major problem in hospitals. While there is no way of proving how many patients die from it, the fact remains that most of them are in a weakened condition in the first place. It is not unreasonable to assume that malnutrition may cause or hasten their demise.

When a large Boston hospital tested surgical patients for protein and calorie malnutrition, half of them were not getting enough of either one. A quarter of the patients were sufficiently malnourished to lengthen their hospital stay. Other studies have discovered malnutrition in from one-quarter to one-half of the patients in hospitals. It is a common cause of death among elderly patients.

The hazards of being in a hospital should cause any person, man or woman, to think at least twice before entering one, except for emergency treatment of injuries or in situations that are demonstrably a matter of life and death. Certainly it is folly to go to the hospital to have a baby, or even for treatment of any disease that can be dealt with at home. Comparative studies show that even patients who suffer severe heart attacks fare no better when they are admitted to the hospital than they do when they are treated at home.

The safety and quality of hospitals varies greatly, of course, but that is not to say that any of them are very good. The point is moot, in any event, because patients who are sent to them are rarely given an opportunity to make an informed choice. Women who wouldn't think of visiting a vacation resort without thoroughly checking it out must accept the hospital of their doctor's choice. That's not true of the nurses who work in them, though. One group of 10,000 nurses was questioned about hospital preferences and a third of them said they would refuse admission to the hospitals in which they worked. Presumably they knew full well what would be done to them there. The same nurses weren't very enthusiastic about the medical attention provided in hospitals, either. More than 40 percent reported seeing doctors make errors that resulted in the patient's death.

I have tried, in this chapter, to alert you to some of the reasons for avoiding hospitals. I'll conclude by warning you to be very skeptical of the excuses your obstetrician will give for sending you there. The complications that a pregnant woman is told to fear are rarely a hazard when the baby is delivered at home. Most of them are real, all right, but they occur only because of the things the obstetrician does to the mother in the hospital after she gets there.

One complication that the doctor is sure to warn you about is the possibility that your baby will have the umbilical cord wrapped around its neck. He will tell you that this can kill your baby in a matter of minutes, so he must have you in the hospital where he can deal with the problem in time. What he doesn't tell you is that it is very common for the baby to have the cord wrapped around its neck, and that it is not inherently dangerous, whether it is wrapped around once, twice, or several times. However, it can be a serious complication when it occurs in the hospital where there has been induced labor, profuse analgesia and anesthesia, and other intervention, and the cord has been unduly compressed. It is not a good reason for going to the hospital, but it is a very good reason for having your baby at home.

The same principle holds for most of the other hazards your doctor will use to frighten you. A prolapsed cord is not uncommon in hospital deliveries because the doctor ruptured the membranes, but it rarely happens in births at home. Hemorrhage—another complication your doctor will point to—often occurs in the hospital because of premature delivery of the placenta and for other reasons, but it rarely occurs in the more relaxed environment of your home.

Your doctor will probably refer to the unsanitary conditions in your household and use that as an excuse to send you to the most unsanitary facility to be found. He will tell you that there isn't enough technology in your home to monitor your labor properly, when in fact it is the inaccuracy of the fetal monitoring equipment in the hospital that provides him with many excuses to intervene needlessly. He will say that there isn't adequate personnel at home. That may sound reasonable unless you know that the multiple vaginal examinations you will receive from the cadre of doctors, nurses, and students in the hospital often produce a pathology of their own.

I don't expect you to debate the specifics of home-versus-hospital risk with your doctor, of course. However, when he tries to dissuade you from having your baby at home by offering a host of insupportable arguments, you might throw some *facts* at him. Ask him to explain the report by Dr. Lewis E. Mehl, of the University of Wisconsin infant development center, who studied 2,000 births, nearly half of them at home, and found striking differences. For example:

- There were 30 birth injuries among the hospital-born babies and none among those born at home.
- 52 of the babies born in the hospital needed resuscitation, against only 14 of those born at home.
- 6 hospital babies suffered neurological damage, compared to 1 born at home.
- None of the home-born babies died after birth, although the national infant mortality rate is more than 22 per 1,000 births.

Despite the statistical evidence to the contrary, doctors continue to denigrate home births. However, I am pleased to observe that women are beginning to fight back. When an obstetric anesthesiologist wrote to the *Washington Post* to disparage home birth and warn of its hazards, the newspaper got a prompt and firm reply from a woman reader. She wrote that taking the opinion of an obstetric anesthesiologist about natural, home birth was like "taking the opinion of an oil magnate on the value of solar energy." She went on to point out that of 420 home births in the District of Columbia there was only one infant mortality, and even that one was not due to a birth complication.

You can't find decent overall statistics on home-versus-hospital birth in the United States because, I suspect, no one wants to collect them for fear of what they will find. What would be found is fairly obvious if you look at the situation in the British Isles, where they *do* collect such statistics and where home birth is the norm. A British report on perinatal mortality released in 1964 showed an overall mortality rate in hospitals that was more than double the mortality rate of babies born at home.

The interest in natural, home birth is growing so rapidly that the obstetricians and the hospitals know that they are in trouble. They are fighting back with a cosmetic approach that provides "birthing rooms" with a homelike atmosphere within the hospital environment. Unfortunately, the cozy atmosphere simply masks the fact that the obstetricians are still doing business in the same old and indefensible way. A wolf in sheep's clothing may *look* less threatening, but he still bites.

American obstetrical practice is the centerpiece of my contention that Modern Medicine is so crisis-oriented that it will invent a crisis if none exists. Almost every stage of obstetrical procedure in the hospital is part of the mechanism that enables the doctor to create his own pathology. Once he has created the pathology, he has his excuse to intervene.

Tragically, it doesn't end there. The complications produced by the intervention often set the woman up as a candidate for the obstetrician's gynecological practice for the rest of her life.

Stay out of the hospital if you can, and if you must enter one, don't allow yourself to be intimidated by your doctor or anyone else. You have a right to know what is being done to you and to be treated with consideration and respect. Ask to see the Patient's Bill of Rights supplied to all hospitals by the American Hospital Association. It says you are entitled to complete, current information on your diagnosis, treatment, and prognosis, and that you have the right to refuse treatment if you desire. That includes the right to reject any or all of the obstetrical interventions that the following chapters describe.

15

"You'll Be Okay; Just Leave Everything to Me."

Women would find having babies a lot less painful, risky, and demeaning if the obstetrical specialty were simply abolished. Except for a handful of doctors who encourage natural birth, obstetricians are guilty of perpetuating an unhealthy, unscientific medical disgrace. As you know by now, I have a low regard for Modern Medicine in general, but obstetrics sets my teeth on edge. It is the only medical specialty in which almost *everything* that the doctor does is medically indefensible and terribly wrong.

I said earlier that doctors have converted pregnancy—a natural, normal, inspiring physiological event—into a nine-month disease. This sounds like a radical concept until you explore the machinations that preceded the creation of the medical specialty.

Throughout most of human history babies were delivered by their mothers, not by doctors, with a female relative or a midwife standing by. Midwives still assist most mothers in many of the most advanced nations in the world. Their success, in terms of infant and maternal mortality, surpasses that of American obstetricians, who have distorted childbirth with ritual procedures that endanger both mother and child. Obstetricians also deny mothers and fathers the joy that natural childbirth should provide.

American obstetrical practice is flawed because its roots are not in medical science, but in historical nonsense, male ego, and plain, old-fashioned greed. It originated in Europe, when the eighteenth-century male barber-surgeons realized that they were losing countless opportunities to increase their income and began plotting to take childbirth away from the midwives. It wasn't easy to do, because midwives were quite capable of assisting at childbirth and had been demonstrating this capability for thousands of years. True, maternal and infant mortalities were then tragically frequent, as today's obstetricians are fond of pointing out, but only because Ignacz Semmelweis had not yet demonstrated that infections are caused by germs passed from doctors to mothers. Conveniently forgotten is the fact that maternal and infant death rates doubled when the barber-surgeons got into the act. Hospitalized mothers got childbed fever because the doctors rushed from sick beds and autopsies to deliveries without bothering to wash their hands.

The doctors had no excuse to co-opt childbirth as long as it was perceived as a nonmedical physiological function that mothers could accomplish themselves with little more than emotional support. In order to get their hands on all those patients, the doctors *had* to convert childbirth into a disease. They did it by interfering with the natural process and creating medical interventions that only they could perform. As insurance, they defamed the midwives, branding them as witches when they lost mothers or babies and having them tortured or burned at the stake. The first "witch" hanged in the American colonies was a midwife whom the doctors accused.

A landmark event in the doctors' long campaign to take over childbirth was the invention of the forceps by Peter Chamberlen in 1588. He and three generations of his family won acclaim for handling difficult deliveries by using a primitive version of this now abused and overused tool. They kept the device a secret from other doctors—and from mothers, too—by working under a sheet and carrying their forceps around in a locked wooden box. This instrument was the obstetricians' first leap into technology, hailed by them as proof of their superiority over the midwives. No one kept score on how often it mangled soft, tiny heads. Chamberlen set a pattern for technological intervention—and for its adverse consequences—that dominates obstetrical practice in the United States today. Obstetricians should build him a shrine and pay him homage every time they go to the bank.

The forceps, however, was not the obstetrical breakthrough that finally took the process of childbirth away from the midwives—and from mothers, as well. The turning point was the elimination of the birthing stool, on which mothers delivered babies by allowing natural contractions and gravity to do their work. Doctors began placing mothers flat on their backs on high tables, with their knees raised. This made it virtually impossible for them to deliver their own babies and assured that they would need a doctor to help.

The supine lithotomy position is the basis for most of the intervention that is routine in modern obstetrical practice. It has effectively deprived women of all control over their childbirth experience. It has also made having babies infinitely more difficult, perilous, and painful, and provided obstetricians with countless seemingly rational reasons to come to the mother's aid. As a doctor once commented in *The Journal of Pediatrics,* obstetricians are like firemen. They both rescue people—the only difference is that *the firemen don't start their own fires!*

Considering the radical nature of the change from the birthing stool to the supine position, you would assume that it evolved from cautious scientific research. Incredibly, it didn't. *The practice of laying birthing mothers flat on their backs was initiated to satisfy a kinky erotic aberration of France's Louis XIV!*

King Louis, it seems, got his kicks by peering from behind a curtain while his mistresses, of whom there were many, gave birth. He was frustrated because his vision was obscured when the women were seated on birthing stools. In an inspired moment he used his royal clout to persuade a male midwife to improve his view. A woman was placed on a high, flat table, with her knees up, and King Louis was immensely pleased with the result.

Not surprisingly, other doctors soon concluded that what was good enough for the royal household must also be good for everyone else. They adopted the lithotomy position, apparently in the belief that Newton and Kepler were wrong, and that by royal edict the law of gravity had been repealed.

That episode might be amusing as a footnote to medical history were it not for the continued use of this ridiculous position by obstetricians delivering babies today. The only refinement that has been added is one that Louis himself might have appreciated but that mothers certainly don't—the use of stirrups that keep the mother's legs strapped in place. The lithotomy position can't be defended for any reason other than the doctor's convenience. From the mother's agonizing perspective the delivery could be made more difficult only if she were hung up by her heels.

Way back in 1933 Mengert and Murphy, in an extensive experimental study, recorded intra-abdominal pressure at the height of maximum straining effort during labor. Their research involved more than 1,000 observations of women placed in seven postures. They found that the greatest pressure was exerted in the sitting position. This was due to measured visceral weight and to increased muscular efficiency. In 1937, another researcher presented x-rays and measurements that indicated that squatting alters the pelvic shape in a way that makes it advantageous for delivery. I know of no study that has ever negated this evidence that women should not be confined to the supine position during labor. Yet with few exceptions, women in labor in the United States are still placed flat on their backs with their feet in stirrups.

Since it obviously has no legitimate medical basis, you are entitled to ask why doctors continue to force mothers to have their babies while strapped down flat on their backs. In the absence of any other rational explanation, I will give you the only answer that makes any sense. The position itself creates the pathology that makes normal births abnormal and provides the obstetrician with about 95 percent of his reason to exist. The trauma that the doctor has *created* provides him with a succession of opportunities to appear necessary and to satisfy his desire to intervene. Meanwhile, the mother has become a bit player in the drama of her own child's birth, and the father is lucky if he is even allowed to be one of the props in the scene.

The pregnant woman's troubles often begin even before she enters the hospital. Although she and her husband may have violated the speed limit to get there because her contractions were frequent and strong, they often slow down abruptly—or even stop—the moment she walks up to the hospital door. This reaction is so common that it even has a name—uterine inertia—and those who have studied it believe it is the result of *fear.*

When she enters the hospital, the mother's apprehension escalates because she immediately loses the support of her husband. She is placed in a wheelchair and trundled off to the labor room, leaving her husband behind at the admission desk. He can't go with her because he is needed for the hospital's most important rite—assuring the business office that he will be able to pay the bill.

Any doctor who is not blinded by his own training and prejudices knows that labor is prolonged and made more difficult and painful by fear. I have had the pleasure of observing—even in my own daughters—the relaxed, rewarding experience that an undrugged natural home birth can be. Fear is neutralized by comfortable, familiar surroundings and the support and comfort of family and friends. Yet virtually every aspect of modern obstetrical practice conspires to isolate the mother in unfamiliar surroundings and increase her apprehension.

The labor room to which the mother is sent has all the appeal of a prison cell, and for all practical purposes that is what it becomes. The typical bare, dismal cubicle is scarcely large enough to contain a metal washstand and a hospital bed. Separated from her husband, the mother stands there frightened and alone, obeying commands from an overworked and often indifferent and impatient nurse. She is told to strip and slip into an ill-fitting hospital gown that ties with strings and flops open in the back, doing nothing to improve her morale. Then she is ordered to climb into bed.

That seemingly innocuous act seals her fate, for until she is moved to the delivery room she will be confined to her bed. She will be denied the freedom of movement and exercise that would relieve her tensions, ease her fears, expedite her labor, and reduce or eliminate her pain. Her baby will be exposed to the risk of damage or death from lack of nutrition and oxygen that the supine position may cause, and the hazards that will result from its mother's treatment with drugs.

The mother's pain will be increased, so drugs will be administered that will retard and prolong her labor. Labor will be induced by invading the uterus and rupturing the membranes, increasing the risk of infection and fetal damage or death. The mother will be further confined by attachment of intravenous gadgetry to keep a vein open for administration of drugs and to provide nourishment because she will not be allowed to eat or drink. A fetal monitor will be strapped to her abdomen, or inserted into her uterus and *screwed into the baby's scalp,* to monitor the fetal trauma that the obstetrician's intervention may well induce. Ultimately, and usually for the convenience of the doctor, oxytocin will be administered to expedite labor, resulting in tetanic (and titanic) contractions so strong that they may injure the fetus. The mother's pain, which escalates because of the way she is being treated, becomes so unbearable that pain-killing injections are given that paralyze the lower half of her body. The mother can no longer feel her contractions and must be told when to push.

Finally, the poor woman is moved to the delivery room, strapped into stirrups, and an episiotomy is performed. The *doctor* delivers the baby because the mother is no longer able to do it, and more often than not he will use forceps because he is unwilling to wait for nature to take its course.

Thus concludes the mother's experience with the "miracle of birth."

The doctor hurriedly cuts the cord before it has stopped pulsating, so the infant's blood backs up in the mother. It is that mixing that produces erythroblastosis (Rh disease) in a subsequent child. He tugs on the cord to expedite delivery of the placenta, increasing the mother's risk of hemorrhage and possibly leaving some pieces behind. He must then invade the uterus to capture the fragments. The mother's risk of infection, already increased over the previous hours by multiple vaginal examinations, becomes even greater. Next, he must repair the damage done to the perineum by the episiotomy he performed. As I will explain later, this may cause sexual dysfunction later on.

Finally, in denial of everything that prompted the mother to go through this ordeal, the baby is whisked off to the newborn nursery, and the mother to the recovery room to sleep off the drugs.

This is motherhood?

This is medicine?

16

"Now Let's Make You Nice and Clean for the Baby."

Translated, that means, "We're going to give you an unpleasant and demeaning enema you don't need, and shave off your pubic hair, even though it may cause an infection that will make you sick."

Why are they done? Few things in this world happen without some kind of reason. There are sound medical reasons why these events shouldn't transpire, so there must be more obscure reasons why they do. I will give you three choices.

1. *Obstetricians are idiots.* Granted, but they can't *all* be idiots. Yet these procedures are routine in hospital births.

2. *Obstetricians can't or don't read.* Granted, again, but *some* of them must have read the studies showing that shaving is dangerous. They go back to the early 1930s, and one was done as recently as 1978. The conclusion? Shaving *triples* the danger of maternal infection and is worthless in keeping the mother clean.

3. *These acts help to render the mother defenseless.* The indignity of losing control of her bowels and parting with her pubic hair reduces the mother's strength to resist the even more awesome and dangerous interventions that will follow and also help put the hospital and the doctor totally in charge.

Take your pick.

17

"This Device Will Help Protect Your Child."

Obstetricians have a standard argument they use to frighten a mother into accepting their life-threatening interference in the natural process of birth. They tell her it is needed because the most dangerous trip her baby will take in its lifetime is the journey through the birth canal. That is utter nonsense if natural birth is permitted, but I will agree that the trip is a risky one, indeed, if there is an obstetrician at the wheel.

I read a fascinating report the other day about a doctor who used a fiberoptic endoscope to light the interior of a woman's uterus so he could take a fetal blood sample. It fascinated me because it seems to support my view that some doctors have less sense than an unborn child.

The doctor wrote that after inserting the fetoscope into the mother's uterus he "had the blood vessel lined up and was just about to strike when out of nowhere came this hand to knock away the needle. I think it was coincidental," he said, "but who knows?"

Who knows, indeed. Obviously, the baby couldn't have known about the risks of fetoscopy, but considering the dangers it poses, the baby's actions made more sense than the doctor's did. The procedure he was using can cause fetal death, leakage of amniotic fluid later in pregnancy, uterine bleeding, scarring of the uterus, infection, puncture of other organs, and psychiatric disturbances. Those are consequences that have actually been observed. In addition, there is the possibility of damage to the eyes of the fetus from the intense light—a hazard that has yet to be studied adequately.

Medical technology is fast overtaking the appliance manufacturers in producing new gadgets that society could very well do without. The difference is that a new hot dog cooker may damage a wiener or two, but gadgetry like the fetoscope can damage both mother and child. How do you forgive a doctor who uses new, unproven medical technology to experiment on a mother or child?

Perhaps the most senseless application of medical technology is the use of electronic fetal monitors in a steadily growing percentage of normal hospital births. It is estimated that between 50 and 75 percent of all hospital births are already being monitored, and a U.S. Senate subcommittee found that in six large Washington hospitals the rate has already reached 100 percent.

Fetal heart monitors were originally developed for use in the approximately 5 percent of pregnancies that are considered high risk. The world-famous obstetrician who developed them, Dr. Roberto Caldeyro-Barcia, is among those who deplore the indiscriminate way in which they now are used. There are two basic types of monitors—internal and external—that pose some common hazards. Each type of monitor also poses risks of its own.

The external monitor consists of two bands that are strapped around the mother's abdomen and connected to a monitoring unit that records the device's findings on tape. One band is pressure sensitive and measures the strength and frequency of her contractions. The other employs ultrasound to determine the condition of the fetus. The theoretical purpose is to determine whether the fetus is suddenly in distress during labor, making it necessary for the doctor to intervene.

The internal monitor looks like a plastic drinking straw that has been wired for sound. The electrodes run through the tube and terminate in a tiny corkscrew at its end. This monitor is inserted through the mother's vagina into the uterus, where it penetrates the amniotic sac. If the doctor doesn't miss and hit something else, *the corkscrew is twisted into the baby's scalp.*

The first of the hazards common to both types of monitors, which I have already mentioned briefly, is the distressing fact that the mother must lie virtually motionless, flat on her back, to ensure the most accurate readings. In addition to retarding labor and making it more painful, this position interferes with the supply of nutrition and oxygen to the fetus, which can cause brain damage and, in some instances, death. This occurs because the weight of the uterus and the fetus causes occlusion of the common iliac artery. The blood supply to the placenta is reduced, making it less capable of providing oxygen and nourishment to the fetus during the critical hours before birth.

A West German scientist, Albert Huch, measured what happened to the baby's oxygen supply when the mother was kept on her back during labor. Within two minutes the fetal oxygen dropped to the danger point, and it took ten to twelve minutes to get it back to normal with vigorous exercise. Monitored mothers don't get the exercise. I am convinced that the high incidence of learning disabilities, hyperactivity, and similar problems observed in children in the United States is the result of fetal oxygen deprivation that doctors cause during labor.

As I suggested previously, the mothers suffer, too, when they are not allowed to sit up, stand, and walk around during labor. A controlled study of more than 300 women conducted by Dr. Caldeyro-Barcia in 1978 found that labor is shortened, forceps are needed less frequently, and mothers experience less pain and fewer complications if they are not confined to bed and delivered while lying on their backs. In addition, the cervix dilates much more rapidly during the first stage of labor and labor is 25 percent shorter. It is 36 percent shorter for women experiencing their first delivery.

Studies have shown that women who are monitored receive three times as many vaginal examinations as those who are not. They are performed by a succession of nurses, interns, and residents, and they greatly increase the chances that the mother will suffer from infection after her child's birth. The infection rate has been shown to be about three times higher.

The third major defect common to both types of monitors is their disgraceful inaccuracy. Investigators of external monitors find that they fail to produce accurate results from 44 to 63 percent of the time. I wonder whether the doctors who rely on them would keep on using an automobile that failed to work three days out of five.

Internal monitors are more accurate, but they, too, produce false results. They sometimes identify normal heart rates as fetal distress. Perhaps that is not surprising in the face of experiments that prove you can get brain wave readings by inserting electrodes into a bowl of lime gelatin.

External monitoring also is prone to false identification of fetal distress. In addition, it may also yield normal readings when a fetus is actually in distress. This is because it sometimes vibrates in a frequency that makes low heart rates double and cuts high ones in half, making both conditions appear normal.

There are three major consequences of this inaccuracy if the doctor relies on the monitor and acts on its results. He may fail to intervene when needed, because a dying fetus has been made to appear well. He may induce labor and rush to deliver the baby before the cervix is sufficiently dilated to permit an easy natural birth. Or—and this is the gravest hazard of all—the doctor may perform a needless Caesarean section in order to deliver a perfectly healthy mother of a perfectly healthy child.

Dr. Albert D. Havercamp, head of the high-risk obstetrics section at Denver General Hospital, says that the use of internal fetal monitors nearly doubled the number of Caesarean sections performed in American hospitals between 1971 and 1976. He maintains, on the basis of studies he has conducted, that the use of the devices has not improved the infant mortality rate, infant performance on the physiological tests performed immediately after birth, or the infants' neurological condition. "I really believe we are in danger of overselling our technology," he declared.

"Oversell" is certainly a well-chosen word. There is obviously a lot of profit for the doctor when a false monitor reading results in a Caesarean and raises the cost of the delivery from approximately $700 to about $3,000!

Even when the monitors record accurate readings there is a significant possibility that the obstetrician won't be able to interpret the results correctly. Dr. Richard Paul of the University of Southern California noted that physicians now administering the tests often lack the necessary training to conduct and interpret them properly. He compared their use of the monitors to the risks of allowing a ten-year-old to drive a car!

Dr. W. R. Jarzembski, professor of biomedical engineering at Texas Technical University, complained in an article that he is often asked to develop designs that are "idiot proof." He said it made him wonder if in so doing he is raising a generation of idiots. Then he pointed out a crucial factor in the indiscriminate use of monitors:

> Medical support personnel may develop an overreliance on the monitoring devices with an attendant lack of personal attention to the patient. Personal attention may have more therapeutic value than the gathering of information by the monitor.
>
> Will medical support personnel become more proficient in the operation of machines only to become less proficient with their knowledge of the needs of the patient?

My answer to his question is, "Yes. They not only will; they already have."

Each of the two types of monitors also poses some specific dangers that are uniquely its own. The external monitors, which use ultrasound to penetrate the mother's body and produce sound waves that measure the condition of the fetus, may pose risks that have yet to be revealed. In 1978 the FDA estimated that they were being used on a million women a year, although the devices have not been declared safe through rigorous testing. Researchers at the FDA Bureau of Radiological Health, noting independent studies revealing harmful effects from ultrasound, said more study is needed before the safety of the procedure can be determined.

In 1973 a study revealed changes in amniotic fluid that had been exposed to ultrasound. Of 65 amniotic fluid specimens taken from patients who had been exposed to ultrasound, 35 (60 percent) failed to grow on culture media. Only 13 of 106 specimens (12 percent) obtained from patients who had not been exposed failed to grow. Investigators also have found delayed neurological development, altered emotional and behavioral effects, fetal abnormalities, and blood and vascular changes in animals exposed to ultrasound.

The risks inherent in internal monitoring have been more clearly established than those that accompany the external type. The amniotic sac must be ruptured prematurely in order to attach the monitor. This disposes the fetus to cord accidents and also denies it the protection of the surrounding amniotic fluid during labor. As a result, damage may be done to the baby's head and unnecessary pressure may be placed on its brain, which could lower the infant's potential IQ.

Other complications, in the form of accidents and infections, may also ensue from the attachment of the monitor to the baby's scalp. A scalp rash from the electrode occurs in 86 to 99 percent of newborns. Many infants subsequently develop scalp abscesses, which may cause permanent bald spots, osteomyelitis, or generalized infection and death. Accidents that have been noted include broken points that require surgical removal, placing of the sharply pointed electrode in the baby's eye, genitalia, or other parts of its body, piercing of the brain, dislodgement of the electrode with subsequent hemorrhage, and fetal death due to hemorrhage from a blood sampling site—a procedure that is sometimes performed.

The National Center for Health Services Research studied the medical literature on electronic fetal monitoring and offered the following summary of risks versus benefits.

1. The benefits are contradictory and confined to a small decrease in mortality among high-risk patients, particularly low-birth-weight babies.

2. Electronic fetal monitoring results in doubling the rate of Caesarean sections performed.

3. The risk is substantial because its use will result in more infants with respiratory distress syndrome, will cause more fetal and maternal morbidity (illness), and will subject the mother to increased risk of death.

4. The technique costs the country an extra $400 million a year.

Much of legitimate medical practice involves the weighing of benefits against risks, explaining the trade-off to the patient, and employing the treatment with her consent if the benefits outweigh the risks. In the case of routine electronic fetal monitoring, the patient is rarely consulted about its use, and there is no evidence that the benefits exceed the risks.

Investigators at the University of Southern California and at Beth Israel Hospital in Boston analyzed 70,000 deliveries and found no difference in outcomes between monitored and unmonitored infants. Randomized clinical trials have also shown that the use of fetal monitors is unwarranted in normal pregnancies. Even in high-risk pregnancies its use produces outcomes that are no better than those obtained by auscultation of fetal heart tones with a stethoscope and careful attention from the nursing staff.

Perhaps it is time to listen to Senator Edward F. Kennedy, who, as chairman of the health subcommittee of the U.S. Senate, held hearings on fetal monitoring. At their conclusion he urged further study of monitoring risks. He said:

The time to find out is before millions of children are exposed. Otherwise, we are playing Russian roulette with the health of our children.

18

"I Want to Make You As Comfortable As Possible."

"Comfortable" is Modern Medicine's euphemism for "tractable." The obstetrician's benign assurance that he is going to make the mother comfortable is the prelude to the obstetrical version of chemical warfare. The patient is about to become the target of a barrage of analgesics and anesthetics that will be fed to her, dripped into her veins, and jabbed into half a dozen locations, including her cervix and her spine. As they relieve the pain that the doctor's intervention—especially the supine position—is causing, they will also relieve the mother of the capacity to make conscious, rational decisions or to protest what is being done to her.

She should protest, because every drug she is given threatens to injure or even kill her or her child.

Accurate national figures aren't available, but it is estimated that 95 percent of all births in U.S. hospitals are medicated to some degree. Although doctors would have you believe otherwise, the use of drugs in labor and delivery also appears to be increasing. A Houston study found that in 1977 the average mother received 19 different drugs during her pregnancy and delivery. In contrast, pregnant women received an average of only 3.6 drugs in 1963.

Most doctors blame the victim for their use of drugs. They maintain that they administer analgesics during labor and anesthetics during delivery only in response to the needs and demands of the mother. My own observation tells me that they sedate the mother for their own convenience. The mothers would be better off if the obstetricians anesthetized themselves!

In most cases pain so acute that it requires drugs is the result of obstetrical intervention. In a well-managed natural childbirth the mother experiences relatively moderate pain. Certainly it is not at a level that would cause her to use drugs that might injure her child.

However, you don't have to rely on my observations. Dr. Yvonne Brackbill, a professor at the University of Florida and a leading authority on the use of drugs in pregnancy, has come to the same conclusion. She says that "mothers do not receive adequate information on adverse drug reactions, on differences among drug risks, or on alternatives to drugs for relief from pain. The studies also indicate that women have little voice in deciding which if any drugs they will consume."

Dr. Walter Brown of the Harvard Medical School says that the quantity of drugs prescribed during labor is not related to the mother's demands or needs. Instead, it is determined by the doctor's interpretation of the psychological state of the mother, which he makes at about the seventh month of pregnancy.

Obstetrical medication is simply another example of Modern Medicine's "what can be done will be done" syndrome. Even though they know that *all* drugs can be harmful to both mother and child, obstetricians use them freely during labor, rather than taking the time to provide the conditions and the "vocal anesthesia" that can make childbirth so nearly painless that drugs are not required. They know that drugs will keep the mother quiet, make unlimited intervention possible, and allow the doctor to deliver the baby at a time most desirable for him.

Although many doctors give the mother the false assurance that "this drug won't reach your baby," every doctor knows that almost any drug he gives her will cross the placenta and affect the fetus. Yet the typical hospitalized mother gets tranquilizers, sedatives, caudals, epidurals, saddle blocks, paracervical blocks, spinals, and even general anesthetics. There is ample evidence that this may produce physical and intellectual damage to the baby, who is ill prepared to deal with the chemicals that are transmitted from its mother.

Even a full-term, healthy newborn baby is not fully developed at the time of its birth. The brain continues to develop for nearly five years after birth, and drugs received before birth can adversely affect that development. The liver, needed for the metabolism of toxic materials, and the kidneys, which excrete them, are also not fully developed and do not function as effectively as they do in adults. Thus, the newborn infant is incapable of dealing effectively with the drugs that have crossed the placenta and entered its bloodstream during labor and delivery.

More than thirty-five studies have been done of healthy full-term babies whose mothers experienced normal pregnancies but were treated with drugs and anesthetics. Dr. Brackbill, who analyzed their results, told a Senate subcommittee in 1978 that "almost all have found statistically significant behavioral effects of obstetric medication. Furthermore, the direction of these effects is uniformly, without exception, toward behavioral degradation and interference with normal function. NO study has ever demonstrated or even suggested that obstetric medication improves normal functioning."

Dr. Brackbill and an associate analyzed the results of a survey of more than 50,000 children conducted by the National Institutes of Health in the 1950s. They picked the 3,500 healthiest babies whose mothers had received drugs during labor and found the same adverse results.

Doctors who use drugs in pregnancy are prone to ignore the fact that children and adults do not respond in the same way to drugs. They point to physiological evaluation of the newborn, done immediately after birth, and insist that the results prove that the drugs they use are safe. They won't tell you that physiological evaluation of the newborn tells nothing about the long-term effects on the baby of the drugs the mother has received. The behavioral effects, such as underachievement and antisocial behavior in later years, have received almost no investigation. They certainly deserve study, for during the first year of life the effects of obstetric drugs can be seen in the development of the baby's ability to sit, stand, and walk. In later years the effects are observed in the development of language and cognitive skills.

Dr. Alvin J. Ericson, professor of pharmacy for obstetrics and gynecology at the University of Kentucky Medical School at Louisville, explains what happens:

> Any drug which artificially changes the mother's blood chemistry or alters the intrauterine environment can jeopardize the fetus. Any drug which stops or slows labor or interferes with normal oxygenation of the fetus by shortening the recovery intervals between uterine contractions or by increasing the length and intensity of the contractions beyond the physiologically normal range can damage the fetal brain.

The analgesics, such as Demerol, that are given to the mother in the early stages of labor do more than kill pain. They also affect other mechanisms, including breathing. The mother's brain is relatively resistant to the effects of these drugs, but not so the baby's. It may experience hypoxia (lack of oxygen) as a result of analgesics given to the mother. This threat is compounded by the already present risk of hypoxia due to the supine position in which the mother has been placed. Deprived of an adequate supply of oxygen, the baby may literally try to breathe before it is born in order to gain the oxygen it needs. In so doing, it inhales the amniotic fluid.

Regional anesthetics, such as the paracervical block, may be injected into the mother several times during labor. Studies have shown that this causes severe changes in the fetal heart rate in 35 percent of cases, followed by prolonged acidosis of the fetus. The result is often fetal depression that may have a subsequent effect on the intellectual and motor development of the child. One study showed that the incidence of neurologic depression was three times as great among children of mothers who had paracervical blocks.

The fetal distress produced by drugs is revealed by the fetal monitor if it is working properly. Often this indication causes the obstetrician to perform a Caesarean section that is justified only by fetal symptoms that his indiscriminate use of drugs has produced.

It doesn't have to be that way. Increasingly, determined women are rejecting hospital birth and having their babies comfortably, safely, and pleasantly, at home. There are even a few hospitals where the reckless use of drugs during labor and delivery is being rejected. At the North Central Bronx Hospital in New York, for example, 93 percent of the women are delivered by trained midwives. About 70 percent of the babies score seven or better on the ten-point Apgar measurement of newborn health. Few other hospitals can come close to that.

My mail is filled with horror stories describing the experiences my readers have had with hospitals and obstetricians, but once in a while I get a letter that warms my heart. I'd like to share this one with you:

> My first child was born six months ago, and it was the most exciting experience of my life. Both my husband and I attended natural childbirth classes, and we practiced relaxation and breathing techniques daily. I neither wanted nor received medication during labor, and I felt in control because I knew what was happening and was able to relax and go along with the contractions and labor. My husband's support and my obstetrician's and nurse's encouragement and concern gave me reassurance and strength. It was wonderful to be awake, aware, and helping in the birth of our child and to know she was safe from sedation or possible brain damage from various forms of anesthesia.

Childbirth need not be a pain-filled, frightening time. If you use natural childbirth techniques, have a supportive husband and obstetrician, and use positive thinking, it can be the greatest event of your life.

If Modern Medicine would get out of the way, that is what childbirth could be like.

19

"It's Time to Speed Things Up a Bit."

Most obstetricians resent God's failure to plan childbirth so that they can set fetal office hours and insist that babies arrive between 9 and 5. Many of them remedy this injustice by inducing labor for nonmedical reasons, even though it sometimes means that babies won't be born alive.

There are medical indications for inducing labor in only about 3 percent of births, but you wouldn't know it from the statistics. The National Institutes of Health has found that synthetic oxytocin is used to stimulate labor in about 20 percent of births in the United States and to induce labor in at least 10 percent of them.

The mother is set up for induction of labor shortly after she reaches the delivery room. A bottle of intravenous (IV) fluid is suspended from a stand and attached to a needle placed in a vein in her arm. The arm is then strapped to a board, which prevents the needle from dislodging and also further restricts her ability to move around. The IV will serve two purposes during the interventions that the doctor has in mind. It will partially nourish the mother so that she can be told not to eat. Keeping her stomach empty reduces the danger that she will aspirate vomit if she is given a general anesthetic during the final stages of delivery. The IV also keeps a vein open for the administration of analgesics and of labor-inducing oxytocin later on.

Oxytocin is a natural product of the pituitary gland that is secreted gradually to stimulate labor when a pregnancy is at term. It produces the contractions that expel the fetus from the womb. However, the impatient doctor who wants to deliver the baby when the physician is ready, not when the baby is, doesn't have to wait for the mother's body to produce its own oxytocin. The drug manufacturers have developed synthetic versions—notably Pitocin—that will produce similar results.

Typically, the doctor who decides to induce labor will rupture the amniotic sac early in the first stage of labor. If the second stage of labor doesn't begin within six to eight hours, he will begin administering Pitocin to speed things up. The Pitocin is added to the intravenous fluid so that the mother is often unaware of what is going on.

The procedure is a risky one for several reasons. Natural oxytocin is supplied by the pituitary gland in the amounts needed for the orderly progress of labor. When the doctor stimulates labor he must determine how much Pitocin to use. The patient must be examined frequently, and the dosage must be controlled carefully so that the drug doesn't produce contractions that are too severe, too frequent, and too long. If the dosage is too strong, it can have disastrous consequences for the mother and especially for her child.

Natural rupture of the bag of waters normally occurs at the onset of the pushing stage of labor, when the cervix is fully dilated and ready to permit the baby to be born. Up to that point the fetus is protected from being damaged by the mother's contractions because it is surrounded by the fluid in the amniotic sac. When the doctor ruptures the membranes and releases the amniotic fluid during the first stage of labor, the cervix is usually dilated to only four or five centimeters. The contractions, more severe than normal because of the Pitocin, ram the unprotected head of the fetus against the cervix and bony pelvis. The result can be brain damage and disalignment of the parietal bones. The potential for damage is multiplied if the doctor has misjudged the delivery date and labor is induced while the baby is not fully developed because it is premature.

A second major risk for the fetus is anoxia (lack of oxygen), which can occur for several reasons. Even normal contractions reduce the supply of oxygen to the baby, but there is an adequate recovery period in between them. When the contractions are longer, stronger, and more frequent because labor has been induced, the baby's loss of oxygen is greater, and there is less recovery time in between. As in the case of oxygen loss caused by other drugs, this may result in brain damage, learning disabilities, and psychotic disorders that will become evident later on. Anoxia can also result when the umbilical cord is compressed or descends before the baby is delivered, which often occurs with induced labor—a condition known as a prolapsed cord.

Other hazards of induced labor include malpositioning of the fetus, which makes delivery more difficult; rupture of the uterus; cranial hemorrhage in the baby; maternal hemorrhage after delivery; and Caesarean sections performed because of fetal trauma caused by induced labor. Caesareans feature a host of complications of their own that will be discussed later in this book.

Induced labor also increases the need for Demerol or other pain-killing drugs and exposes mother and baby to the hazards that they produce. A 1975 British study compared 614 mothers whose labor was drug induced with a control group. Half of the noninduced mothers got through labor without any pain-killing drugs. Only 8 percent of the induced mothers did.

The doctor's primary motivation for the induction of labor is his own convenience, not the welfare of the mother or her child. However, he won't admit that; instead, he will blame the victim. He will say that the mother wasn't strong enough to cope with the ordeal of a long labor or that she wasn't able to stand the pain. I have even heard elective induction defended as necessary so that a delivery date could be scheduled and the mother could arrange for a baby-sitter.

If the reasons for inducing labor were valid, one could expect that such interventions would occur at a reasonably stable rate from one hospital to the next. They don't, which confirms that it is the doctors rather than the patients who want labor induced. I have never seen national statistics, but a New Jersey study revealed hospital labor induction rates ranging from a low of .1 percent to a high of 25 percent. Labor was stimulated with drugs at a rate of 3 percent in the lowest case to a high of 71 percent in the hospital that induced labor most often. That institution must have a lot of obstetricians who like to play golf!

In 1978, the Food and Drug Administration cautioned doctors against the elective induction of labor for nonmedical reasons. FDA Director Donald Kennedy said that the use of drugs to induce labor had not been sufficiently tested to guarantee the safety of the child, and that the use of drugs like oxytocin "for the convenience of the doctor and the patient" was inappropriate.

Every mother wants to give birth to a healthy, normal child, equipped with all of the priceless gifts that God intended. Don't count on your obstetrician to give your baby that chance. Make your desire for an undrugged, natural birth clear to him before he slips you some Demerol, or neither you nor your baby will have a fighting chance.

Modern Medicine's meddling with nature is not limited to speeding up deliveries. Sometimes, again for their own purposes, doctors want to slow them down. A doctor who is late for a delivery often advises the labor room nurse, by telephone, to give the mother drugs that will retard labor and tell her to cross her legs and stop pushing until he arrives.

I have known cases in which a doctor knew he wouldn't get to the hospital on time but telephoned to order a general anesthetic for the mother so she wouldn't know he wasn't there. When he reached the hospital he rushed into the delivery room after the nurses had delivered the baby, hurried into a surgical cap and gown, and tied a mask around his neck. After glancing at the somnolent mother, he dashed breathlessly into the waiting room and proudly announced to the father, "Congratulations. It's a boy!"

The mother, if she only knew it, should be grateful to him for not getting there in time because she escaped the episiotomy he would have performed. Instead, she remains eternally grateful to him for the skill with which he delivered her child!

20

"I'm Going to Sew You Up Like a Virgin."

Doctors are hard put to legitimize their role in childbirth. About 95 percent of the time they are as superfluous as tailors in a nudist colony. That is why Modern Medicine has had to distort the process of childbirth to create the pathology that doctors will be needed to treat.

Obstetricians cause the mother pain so that she will need drugs that only doctors can prescribe. They immobilize her so that complications ensue. Then they position her during delivery so that she will need the episiotomy that a doctor must perform. The position creates the need for the surgery, and the need for surgery is then used to justify the position that makes it easier for the surgery to be performed. Once again Modern Medicine looks as foolish as a kitten chasing its tail.

The perineum, through which a baby must pass in order to be born, is a remarkably flexible part of the anatomy. Bodily changes cause it to become even more so during the period before the baby is delivered. If the mother is in a natural

177

position for childbirth and is coached on when to push and when not to push, the baby can usually be eased out without damage to the mother or itself. However, as I have pointed out, the mother is *not* in a natural position for childbirth when an obstetrician is in charge. She is placed on her back with her feet in stirrups so that the baby must be delivered *against* the force of gravity and the upward curve of the pelvis. In this position, the perineum is more likely to tear.

Obstetricians cite the possibility that the perineum may tear as their excuse to perform an episiotomy. This operation is a slashing of the perineum to widen the opening of the vagina so that it will be easier for the baby to emerge. The operation has become so routine that it is performed on about 85 percent of first-time mothers in the United States. Its value must be questioned, however, when you observe that it is rarely performed in countries where natural birth is favored. In Holland, for example, the operation is performed on less than 8 percent of mothers, and in England it is used on only about one in seven.

American doctors use a litany of explanations to rationalize doing the episiotomy. They include:

It must be done for the sake of the baby. There is no evidence that it does anything to spare the baby from harm.

It assures that the perineum won't tear. What logic! Virtually all women have their perineums slashed surgically so a fraction of them won't tear.

The episiotomy heals better than a tear. In fact, the opposite is true.

It will prevent prolapse of the reproductive organs and collapse of the pelvic floor. This argument was reported in a medical text half a century ago as a suspicion that had no scientific basis. No subsequent scientific research supports it, but the assertion is now presented in the current version of the text as a statement of fact.

The operation will return the mother to her virginal state and improve her sex life. It won't. More often it will make her sex life worse.

There are a lot of things obstetricians *don't* tell the mother that she is entitled to know. They don't tell her the following facts:

- Episiotomies require local anesthesia and increase the risk of damage from drugs.
- Occasionally a needle is jammed into the baby's brain when the anesthetic is administered, causing its death.
- The increase in episiotomies has been accompanied by an increase in accidents in which the knife goes too deep and the anal sphincter is slashed.
- The perineum is so flexible that after delivery it will retract to its normal condition even though no episiotomy is performed. Sometimes, in fact, the vaginal muscles will grip more tightly than before.
- When he performs an episiotomy, the doctor cuts through muscles and nerves, producing a numbness that sometimes persists for years.
- The incision is two inches long on the outside and two inches long on the inside, so there are actually *four* inches of incision that stitches must be used to repair.
- Repairing an episiotomy usually takes longer than the delivery itself. Natural tears are likely to be superficial, so only a few stitches are required most of the time.
- The operation increases the risk of postpartum infection and is responsible for about 20 percent of maternal deaths.

All of us want to feel needed, even when we are not. But should women pay with their lives so that obstetricians can feel better about their lot?

21

"Your Pelvis Is Too Small."

When I was a young doctor, an obstetrician whose Caesarean section rate reached 10 percent was a pariah among his peers. Other doctors knew that the operation was dangerous and could be avoided in all but about 5 percent of cases, so the skill of an obstetrician was measured in an inverse ratio to the number of sections he performed.

The maternal death rate from Caesarean sections is still six times that of vaginal deliveries. The rate of postpartum uterine infection is more than fourteen times greater among women who are delivered—as the obstetricians put it—"from above." One-third of the women who have Caesarean sections suffer postoperative hemorrhage or infection, to say nothing of severe abdominal and intestinal pain, exhaustion, and depression. Thus, all of the reasons for avoiding surgical delivery still remain, but one factor has changed. In the 1960s only one baby in twenty was delivered by Caesarean section. In 1979 it was almost one baby in six.

180

The Caesarean section rate in the United States has soared to 15 per-cent—three times the number that can be justified medically—yet doctors point to this sorry record with pride!

This attitude may appear irrational, but it is easy to explain. Doctors learn little or nothing about natural birth in medical school. The emphasis is all on complications and intervention, so doctors are always delighted when they have the opportunity to do what they have been taught to do—intervene. That's why obstetricians have always struck me as the Little Jack Horners of Modern Medicine. The Caesarean section is the plum in their obstetrical pie. The doctor messes up the mother with a succession of reckless procedures, declares an emergency, slices open her belly, and pulls out her baby. When he has finished displaying his surgical talent, the look on his face says, "My, what a good boy am I."

Most of the rituals and technology described in the previous chapters have contributed to the shocking increase in the number of Caesarean sections that are being performed. They are responsible for a whole catalog of creative symptoms, most of them scarcely heard of twenty years ago. All of them are taken as indications for surgical delivery of the baby. The diagnoses include fetal distress, failure to progress, arrested descent, failure to dilate, and God knows what else. Meanwhile, prolonged labor has been redefined. The duration of labor taken as an indication of need for a Caesarean section has dropped progressively from the seventy-two hours that was generally accepted when I began my medical practice. It dropped to forty-eight hours, then twenty-four hours, twelve hours, and now, if the doctor is eager enough, even two hours will do.

If immobilization of the mother, artificial rupture of the membranes, drugs, Pitocin to induce labor, and fetal monitoring all fail to produce a convincing symptom as an excuse for a Caesarean, the doctor always has a last card up his sleeve. He can shake his head sadly and blame the victim by telling the mother that her pelvis is too small to permit the birth of her child.

A previously sectioned mother has long been a sitting duck when another baby is due. "Once a Caesarean, always a Caesarean," has been the medical dictum, although there was ample evidence that this was not true. Ninety-eight percent of mothers who had delivered a previous baby by C-section had the operation again for the birth of their next child, even though the indications were not the same.

It made no difference that in 1963 two doctors at Cornell Medical College had reported that vaginal delivery for women who previously had been delivered from above did not increase maternal mortality. On the contrary, they found that it decreased maternal deaths because it eliminated the hazards of abdominal surgery. Despite this evidence, "Once a section, always a section" remained the conventional obstetric wisdom for another seventeen years.

Not until 1980, after the Caesarean section rate had tripled in the United States, did the National Institutes of Health issue new guidelines telling doctors that vaginal delivery for women who previously had been sectioned is as safe as, or safer than, another section. The guidelines also urged that when labor contractions are not strong enough women be permitted to move around and exercise to stimulate natural labor. Only after exhausting all other measures should surgery be employed.

The new guidelines make some additional recommendations that will probably give obstetricians fits. They recommend against routine use of Caesarean sections for babies in the breech position and urge that hospitals liberalize their policies to allow the baby's father or another relative to be in the operating room when the Caesarean is performed.

I will watch with interest to see what effect the new guidelines have. They didn't tell the obstetricians anything they didn't already know, but they certainly tell mothers some things the obstetricians didn't want them to hear. Perhaps they will persuade the doctors to give their scalpels a rest.

There are many reasons why Caesarean sections shouldn't be performed unless they are absolutely essential to save the life of a mother or child. Besides the risks of complications and death, many women experience adverse psychological effects, and all of them are denied the pleasure that natural childbirth can bring.

The effects of the drugs and anesthetics, coupled with the severe pain and the physical limitations imposed by major surgery, interfere with two other vital elements of motherhood. The bonding that should occur immediately after birth, regarded as essential to the future relationship between mother and child—or even among mother, father, and child—becomes impossible. The baby is whisked off to the newborn nursery because the mother is knocked out by drugs, has an intravenous needle in her arm, and a Foley catheter draining her bladder. Her condition also makes it so difficult and painful to initiate breast-feeding that she often abandons it entirely, which will also adversely affect her child.

The baby may also be affected in other ways. Potential brain damage is already present because of the doctor-induced anoxia that probably brought the mother to the operating room in the first place. In addition, if the doctor was mistaken about the expected delivery date, the baby may be delivered prematurely and bear all of the consequences that prematurity implies. Finally, and perhaps most serious of all, the baby may become the victim of hyaline membrane disease.

This disease is an often fatal lung condition found only in premature babies and babies delivered by Caesarean section. It occurs when excess fluid, normally forced out by the muscular action of the uterus during vaginal delivery, remains in the baby's lungs. There are 40,000 cases of this disease every year, and it is estimated that 6,000 of them could be prevented if doctors didn't induce delivery or perform a Caesarean section before spontaneous labor was well under way and the baby was ready to leave the womb.

Doctors always defend the Caesarean sections they perform as lifesaving measures needed by the mother and child. The statistics alone, of course, give that claim the lie. In addition, however, there are other clear indications that it is the doctor's interests, not the mother's or the baby's, that are served when Caesareans are performed.

Back in the 1960s, obstetrics was one of the lowest-paid

medical specialties, although in 1963 there were 261 live births for each obstetrician, creating the opportunity for each of them to deliver a baby every working day. Because of the increase in the number of obstetricians, and the declining birth rate, the situation changed radically by 1975. In that year the number of live births per doctor was only 145.

Were the obstetrician-gynecologists starving to death? On the contrary. Thanks to the soaring rate of Caesarean sections and hysterectomies, obstetrics-gynecology had become the highest-paid medical specialty of all!

Another fascinating insight can be gained by examining the hours of the day during which Caesarean sections are performed. If, as the doctors insist, the 546,000 sections performed in 1979 were truly emergencies, one would expect to find them spread rather evenly around the clock. All of the evidence says that they are not.

A curious scientist at Johns Hopkins University in Baltimore studied 123 births to determine the hours during which they occurred. There were twenty *emergency* Caesarean sections among these births. For some curious reason sixteen of these "emergencies" occurred during the daylight hours, between 8:00 A.M. and 7:59 P.M. Only four of the Caesarean sections were performed during the twelve nighttime hours when the doctors preferred to be home in bed.

Dr. Andrew Fleck, director of New York state's Division of Maternal and Child Health, found a similar discrepancy in 1978. He studied first-time Caesareans and found that 62 percent of them occurred during normal working hours, and only 38 percent between 6 P.M. and 7 A.M. He also found that C-section rates varied from a low of 2 percent to a high of 22 percent in different hospitals in the state of New York.

"What we've been able to show is that Caesarean section is a provider attitude and not an attribute of the women," Dr. Fleck said in an interview. "If you go to a doctor who likes to do Caesarean sections, you're going to get sectioned. In other words, snakebite poisoning is a function of the kind of snake that bites you."

If you want to avoid snakebite, have your baby at home.

22

"It's a Boy!"

I can remember a time when Americans were appalled by tales about the ancient Chinese custom of throwing female babies into the Yangtze River. Modern Medicine has now developed its own version of this incredible custom, but it doesn't seem to bother the doctors who use it at all. The process is known as amniocentesis. It involves inserting a needle into the amniotic sac and withdrawing fluid that contains cells discarded by the fetus. When they are subjected to chromosomal analysis, the cells will reveal fetal deformities and also the sex of the child.

The ostensible purpose of the procedure is to determine whether the fetus will be a victim of Down's syndrome or some congenital abnormality. If the finding is positive, the mother can abort the baby and avoid having a deformed child. Amniocentesis for this purpose is most often used on women over age forty, particularly those who have previously given birth to an abnormal child. At that age, the chances of having a Down's syndrome baby are on the order of 6 percent.

Use of the procedure is growing but is not yet widespread. It was performed on about 25,000 hospital patients in 1978, but that figure doesn't mean much because there is no data on how often amniocentesis is performed on outpatients or in doctors' offices.

The risks of amniocentesis are considerable for both mother and child. It doubles the rate of spontaneous miscarriage and of fetal abnormalities such as respiratory distress syndrome, pneumothorax (air in the baby's chest) from multiple puncture wounds, orthopedic problems, and gangrene of a limb. The mother may experience infection, bleeding, possible mixing of her own and the baby's incompatible blood types, premature rupture of the membranes during pregnancy, and postpartum hemorrhage. There is also sufficient incidence of false positive findings to cause a significant number of abortions of normal babies.

Although most doctors will deny it, there is considerable evidence that many parents seek amniocentesis not to determine fetal abnormalities, but to determine sex. Their intention, of course, is to abort the baby if it is not of the sex they prefer, and there isn't much chance that the aborted baby will be a boy. In fact, qualified medical observers tell me that in abortions performed after amniocentesis, girls are aborted in four cases out of five.

Lately, I have been hearing a standard line from doctors who perform amniocentesis. They say they "performed the procedure for sexual reasons with reluctance." I wonder if they were equally reluctant to collect their $300 to $500 fee?

I don't know where all of the genetic manipulation that is evolving will lead, but amniocentesis troubles me. So does the sexual separation of male sperm cells so that the doctor can do artificial insemination and virtually guarantee that the baby will be a boy.

Feminist Gloria Steinem, in a article in *MS* magazine, fantasized one possibility:

Given the increasing ability to predetermine the baby's sex—

plus the bias toward having more sons and the development of extrauterine birth—the worst of my fantasies passes through decades of decreasing female population, and ends in some zoo of the future with a dozen of us in cages beneath a sign: "Please don't feed the women."

23

"I Know What's Best for Your Child."

A mother is doubly victimized by Modern Medicine. In addition to the abuses *she* suffers, she must also worry about what a doctor may do to her child. Creative diagnosis and the harmful intervention that often follows isn't limited to adults. Doctors will practice it on any available victim, regardless of size.

The damage inflicted on children begins, as noted earlier, when silver nitrate drops are placed in their eyes. It continues throughout childhood in an endless succession of useless examinations, worthless medications, and needless surgery that serve only to make pediatricians rich.

The child's health is often placed at risk shortly after birth when the doctor discourages breast-feeding and urges the mother to raise her baby on formula milk. There is virtually no medical or physical reason, short of a bilateral mastectomy, why doctors should urge substitution of nutritionally deficient formula for a perfect food like mother's milk. Breast-feeding may be impractical for some working mothers, of course, but that doesn't explain why doctors seem so determined to deny the benefits of breast-feeding to all the rest. Many aspects of obstetrical intervention mitigate against breast-feeding and, if these are not sufficient to discourage the mother, pediatricians always seem able to find another excuse. They tell her that her breasts are too small, her milk is too thin, or that she has a cold and should stay away from the baby.

I blame three factors for the failure of doctors to urge that mothers breast-feed their children. First, they learn nothing about nutrition in medical school and are actually taught that formula is just as good as mother's milk. Second, this belief is reinforced by the misleading medical journal advertising purchased by the formula manufacturers. It stops just short of citing women as defective because their breasts aren't calibrated and encased in tin. Finally, I believe doctors oppose breast-feeding for the same reason they oppose natural childbirth. It denies them too many lucrative opportunities to intervene.

Rather than discouraging breast-feeding, conscientious doctors should be doing everything they can to promote it because of its enormous importance to both mother and child. It strengthens the bond between them in a way that no amount of holding and hugging will achieve. It stimulates hormones that reduce postpartum bleeding and discomfort and causes the uterus to contract more rapidly to its normal size. It gives the mother sensual pleasure. It helps protect her from cancer of the breast.

Breast-feeding also stimulates the production of prolactin by the pituitary gland, which enhances maternal behavior. It also has a tranquilizing effect (without drugs) that helps the mother adjust to the pressures of having a new baby in the home. The prolactin also suppresses production by the ovaries of the hormone that triggers ovulation, thus providing natural birth control for a much longer time.

The baby benefits because breast-feeding provides it with nourishment superior to that supplied by formula milk. It provides better bone maturation and intellectual development. It protects the child from asthma and other hereditary allergies. Because nursing babies are not locked into rigid feeding schedules they eat when they are hungry. This makes them less prone to the digestive upsets seen in babies who are allowed to cry until the clock says mother can shove a bottle in their mouths. There is even evidence that the resulting avoidance of emotional disturbances and the breast-fed baby's closer bond to its mother reduce the danger of hypertension later in life.

One of the most important benefits that the baby receives from mother's milk is protection from infectious diseases that the mother has fought off through her well-developed immune system. The bottle-fed baby is much more likely to suffer a nightmare of illnesses that include diarrhea, colic, gastrointestinal and respiratory infections, meningitis, asthma, hives, other allergies, pneumonia, eczema, obesity, arteriosclerosis, dermatitis, growth retardation, hypocalcemic tetany, neonatal hypothyroidism, necrotizing enterocolitis, and sudden infant death syndrome. Babies raised on canned formula milk may also be affected by ingesting too much lead.

Not long ago the American Academy of Pediatrics finally discovered the virtues of breast-feeding and took a strong position in favor of mother's milk. With an enthusiasm usually reserved for products of the pharmaceutical labs, it said that "Human milk is nutritionally superior to formula," and it urged all elements of the medical profession to encourage breast-feeding.

That's mildly encouraging, but I'm not so naive as to believe that the Academy's recommendations will prevail. Hospital personnel don't like breast-feeding because it involves more work for them and upsets their routine. Pediatricians don't like it for the opposite reason. It means less work and fewer office call fees for them. When babies are breast-fed, pediatricians are hard put to justify their existence. There are no diets to juggle and the babies enjoy a natural immunity to most ailments. There's nothing more useless than a doctor who has nothing to treat.

Boy babies, shortly after birth, are subjected to a procedure that is a rare example of worthless intervention that little girls escape. The pediatrician whips out his knife and performs a circumcision—a ceremony that has no legitimacy except as a religious rite. It provides no established medical benefit, is usually done without analgesics before it is safe to do it, and it entails plenty of risks. Next to the usually needless episiotomy performed on women, it is the most frequently performed surgical procedure. Doctors enriched themselves by lopping the foreskin from nearly 1,500,000 penises in 1979. Now and then the knife slipped and, oops! they took the whole thing!

Many obstetricians routinely give vitamin K to newborn babies because they have been taught that infants are born with a deficiency of this vitamin, which influences how quickly blood clots. That's nonsense, unless the mother is malnourished, but doctors do it anyway, and expose babies to another risk. Administration of vitamin K to the newborn may produce jaundice—which gives the pediatrician an excuse to treat it with bilirubin lights. These lights expose the baby to a dozen documented hazards that may require still further treatment and possibly affect the child for the rest of its life.

When the baby escapes from the hospital nursery, the pediatrician still keeps the child on a very short leash. He schedules an extended series of monthly examinations that probably do more harm than good because they provide the doctor with further opportunities to intervene. He will give the baby a series of highly controversial immunizations, telling the mother of the presumed benefits, but never of the risks. If the baby contracts a viral infection it probably will be treated with penicillin, which costs a lot of money but is ineffective against viruses and can't possibly do any good. A child with a cold may be given counterproductive treatments. The pediatrician will prescribe an antihistamine to *dry up* its runny nose and then order a humidifier placed in its room to *moisten* its throat!

It is riskier than Las Vegas to take your child to a pediatrician for treatment of an earache or a mild sore throat. If he is unable to diagnose the sore throat as a strep infection, which can cost you $100 and up, he can always call it tonsillitis and ship the child off to the hospital for a tonsillectomy, which costs even more.

Tonsils have long been the featured attraction in the theater of needless surgery. The star is the surgeon, who is on stage correcting one of God's mistakes. In my lifetime I've watched this act with sorrow as one kid after another—tens of millions of them in the last fifty years—have been lured to the hospital to trade perfectly healthy tonsils for a dish of ice cream.

I don't believe there is more than one case in a thousand in which the tonsils need to be removed. They're in a class of operations that I call "bread and butter" surgery—comparable as a steady income-producer to what tune-ups are for a garage. The difference is that the tune-up costs less, and, when the mechanic gets through with your engine, it probably will run like a top. The prognosis for children who have tonsillectomies is not nearly that good. They risk damage and death, rarely with any beneficial results. The operations cost parents a billion dollars a year, and may actually harm the children who have them since no one really knows what biological functions the tonsils may perform.

In 1965, the tonsillectomy was the most frequently performed surgical procedure in the United States, but the overwhelming weight of scientific evidence against them has caused the number performed to drop significantly. About 1.2 million were performed in 1965, and by 1978, the number had dropped to 548,000.

That's the good news. The bad news is that, in the course of eliminating about half of the needless tonsillectomies, Modern Medicine again confirmed my theory that doctors will never give up one profitable, useless procedure until they have found another equally dubious one to take its place. In this instance the replacement is the tympanostomy, which was performed on 1,173,000 children in 1979.

The tympanostomy is a procedure in which small tubes are inserted through the eardrums to drain the middle ear of children suffering from an infection known as otitis media. It is supposed to prevent hearing loss, but studies indicate not only that it doesn't, but that the operation itself does in some children produce scarring that *causes* hearing loss.

I have barely scratched the surface in this description of pediactric abuses, but to tell the whole story would take another book. It's not going to increase my private practice, but the best advice I can give you as a mother is, "Keep your children away from their pediatricians except in dire emergencies if you want to maintain their health!"

24

"You'll Just Have to Learn to Live with It."

You have probably sensed from the tone of what I've written that my purpose in this book has been to expose the mistreatment of women by their doctors in a way that would elicit an emotional response. I wanted to do more than inform you. I wanted to disgust you, shock you, and frighten you.

I wanted to make you very, very angry!

I hope I have succeeded. I hope I have made you so angry that you'll see your doctor in a new light. The next time you visit him, I hope he will sense from your attitude that he can't treat you as an emotional weakling who is putty in his hands.

I hope you're so disturbed that you'll start asking tough questions when your doctor hands you a prescription, or orders an x-ray, or prescribes a routine test. I want enough women to begin badgering their doctors about their behavior so they'll sense that a revolution is brewing. I want *you* to frighten *them* for a change, to let them know by playing on their most powerful emotion—fear—that their sacrosanct position is threatened.

I hope you're upset enough to defy your doctor and find another one, if necessary, if he insists on dangerous drugs or surgery or other treatment that you and your family don't need. I want you to tell him where *he* can go if he demands that *you* go to the hospital and refuses to deliver your baby at home.

I hope you're angry enough so you won't accept, without careful investigation, a surgeon's compulsion to wield his knife. I want you to think twice and get a second opinion, or as many as necessary, before you submit to a hysterectomy or a mastectomy or a Caesarean section, or any other procedure that may affect you for the rest of your life.

I hope you're so incensed that if you or a member of your family is injured by your doctor—physically or emotionally—you won't "just learn to live with it." I hope you'll hire the best lawyer you can find and sue, sue, sue.

It is my great hope that women will begin resisting the arrogance and ignorance and greed of Modern Medicine so that doctors *won't dare* resist change. I believe you have the power to force them to begin questioning *themselves.* I believe you can cause them to begin doubting the validity of their own medical educations. I believe that you can raise the objections that will compel them to question the integrity and motives of their principal source of continuing education—the drug company detail men and the pharmaceutical ads. I believe you can inspire them, at least the younger ones, to take a new look at their medico-political leadership and at the structure of medical practice in the United States. I believe you may be able to prod them to the point that they'll rediscover the ethics and morality and compassion that prompted their desire to become doctors, but somehow got lost in medical school. Who knows? You may even be able to embarrass them so much that they will become self-conscious about their fees!

Ten years ago I had little hope for my profession. I didn't believe that any power on earth could force a rigid, self-righteous, monopolistic institution like Modern Medicine to change. Today I *know* it can be done. I also know that it is women who will do it because they are the principal victims and they are subjected by their doctors to far more arrogance and condescension than men.

The movement is already underway. I have seen the changes wrought by a small band of intelligent, courageous, determined women who are leading the attack.

Modern Medicine is going to capitulate because of women like you, guided by advocates like Gail Brewer, Lee Stewart, Diana Scully, Doris Haire, Suzanne Arms, Gena Corea, Angela Kilmartin, Barbara Gordon, and victims like Martha Weinman Lear. I urge you to read their works, which are listed in the back of this book.

These exceptional women have already achieved some extraordinary results. They have compelled a change in the blind advocacy by medical leadership of dangerous, ritualistic physical examinations and tests. Breast-feeding has risen from 15 to more than 50 percent. Home birth has tripled in the past two years. The ridiculous "once a section always a section" dogma has been overturned. Women are kicking the habits bestowed on them by their doctor-pushers, and Valium sales are down an estimated 30 percent.

That's only a beginning, but it's an important beginning because it demonstrates that women *do* have the power to effect change. But the generals who are leading the battle need an army.

I hope you'll sign up!

25

Fifty Drugs Every Woman Should Think Twice About Before Taking

We live in an overmedicated society. More Americans are hooked on drugs by their physicians than by all the pushers on the street. It is estimated that one billion prescriptions are written in the United States every year. In my judgment, a majority of them are unnecessary and—as the staff in any hospital emergency room can tell you—many of them are dangerous and even deadly.

Virtually all drugs are toxic in some degree and, as Eli Lilly once said, "a drug without side effects is no drug at all." That is another way of saying that no drug can be pinpointed to affect only the organ it is designed to treat. Most drugs have broad effects and some affect literally every organ system in the body. Some of the side effects are minor nuisances. Others can be severely damaging and even fatal. It is not uncommon for a patient to suffer side effects from a drug that are more discomforting and dangerous than the ailment the drug was supposed to cure.

Information regarding the hazards of every drug is contained in the prescribing information and in the *Physician's Desk Reference* (PDR), which are readily available to your doctor. Unfortunately, many physicians don't bother to study this information, and most of those who do don't bother to share it with their patients. If they did, the patient might refuse to take the drug!

The prudent patient will question her doctor closely about every drug he prescribes. Ask him the name of the drug, why he is prescribing it, and how it works. Ask him when you should take it, how long you should take it, and whether its effectiveness is reduced in association with food. Ask him whether there are any hazards in taking it in combination with other prescription or nonprescription drugs or alcohol. Ask him about the potential side effects and the hazards of overdosage. Ask him what side effects may indicate that you should stop taking the drug, and which of them are serious and should be reported to him.

After answering all of those questions, the doctor may decide not to give you the medication after all. If he still writes a prescription for the drug, go to the public library and look it up in the *Physician's Desk Reference* and compare the side effects he told you about with those listed in the PDR. Then decide whether you want to have the prescription filled.

In the following pages, I have provided information about more than fifty of the drugs that women most frequently ask me about. The trade and generic names are given, followed by the most frequent indications for each drug's use, and some of the listed potential adverse effects you may experience if you take it. Finally, I have added some comments of my own. You are urged, however, to read the complete prescribing information before you take *any* drug.

Aldactone (spironolactone)—Edema (swelling) due to congestive heart failure, hypertension.
> *Adverse effects:* Swelling of the male breast, cramping,
> diarrhea, lethargy, mental confusion, sexual impotence,
> causes tumors in rats.
> *Comment:* Should only be given to patients who have not
> responded to safer antihypertensives.

Aldomet (methyldopa)—Hypertension.
> *Adverse effects:* Fever, fatal liver damage, parkinsonism,
> psychosis, depression, angina, breast enlargement, im-
> potence, decreased sex drive.
> *Comment:* Fatal hemolytic anemia may occur; periodic
> blood counts should be made during therapy.

Aldoril (methyldopa plus hydrochlorthiazide)—Hypertension.
> *Adverse effects:* See Aldomet and Hydrodiuril.

Apresoline (hydralazine)—Hypertension.
> *Adverse effects:* Headache, nausea, vomiting, diarrhea, rapid
> heartbeat, chest pain, tremors, muscle cramps, depres-
> sion, disorientation, anxiety, hepatitis.
> *Comment:* May produce lupus erythematosus. Can cause
> anginal attacks and EKG changes. Should not be used
> during pregnancy.

Atromid-S (clofibrate)—Reduction of cholesterol and serum
lipids.
> *Adverse effects:* Angina, arrhythmias, phlebitis, hair loss,
> gallstones, impotence, weight gain.
> *Comment:* In a large study, there were excessive deaths
> due to malignancy and gall bladder disease in the group
> treated with this drug.

Bendectin (doxylamine plus pyridoxine)—Antinauseant, anti-
emetic.
> *Adverse effects:* Drowsiness, nervousness, stomach pain,
> headache, disorientation.
> *Comment:* A wide variety of fetal skeletal defects and
> other abnormalities have been reported among the
> offspring of mothers using this drug. Many cases are
> now in litigation.

Butazolidin (phenylbutazone)—Arthritis.

Adverse effects: Blood disorders (sometimes fatal); more severe reactions in patients over 40.

Comment: This drug should be avoided by persons with incipient heart failure, blood disorders, pancreatitis, senility, drug allergy, severe kidney and liver disease, history of peptic ulcer.

Clinoril (sulindac)—Arthritis.

Adverse effects: Peptic ulcers, gastro-intestinal bleeding, ear noises, edema.

Comment: Not to be used during pregnancy or nursing.

Dalmane (flurazepam)—Insomnia or frequent awakening.

Adverse effects: Confusion, depression, headache, nausea, constipation, inability to control urination, changes in sex drive, vision problems, liver dysfunction.

Comment: A sleeping pill with side effects that should keep you awake worrying about them. Perhaps it does, because the Academy of Sciences Institute of Medicine says that although 23.5 million prescriptions for sleeping pills were written in 1979, they don't do what they're supposed to do. The Sleep Disorder Clinic at Stanford University has found that 40 percent of insomniac patients actually lost sleep because of sleeping pills. A withdrawal of the medication resulted in 20 percent more sleep. They probably help drug company executives sleep well, though, because the pills bring in an estimated $100 million a year.

Danocrine (danozol)—Endometriosis.

Adverse effects: Acne, hirsutism, decrease in breast size, deepening of voice, oiliness of skin and hair, weight gain, clitoral enlargement.

Comment: The potential masculinizing effects of this drug are so severe that most women will want to avoid it if their doctor can offer an acceptable alternative.

DES (diethylstilbestrol)—Treatment of menopausal symptoms, hormone replacement.

Adverse effects: See Premarin.

Comment: In the early stages of use, DES was prescribed

for repeated miscarriage, use as a "morning-after" pill, and suppression of lactation. Subsequently, it was discovered that the drug sometimes produced vaginal cancer in the female offspring and genito-urinary defects in the male offspring of pregnant women who took it. There is also evidence that the drug may increase the risks of cancer in some postmenopausal women. I subscribe to the view that *all* drugs should be avoided during pregnancy, unless their use is dictated by a life-threatening condition.

Dilantin (phenytoin)—Anticonvulsant (grande mal).

Adverse effects: Slurred speech, mental confusion, twitching, fatal rashes, gum overgrowth, fatal toxic hepatitis.

Comment: Can cause fetal defects if used during pregnancy.

Diamox (acetazolamide)—Edema due to congestive heart failure, petit mal seizures, open angle glaucoma.

Adverse effects: Fever, rash, bone marrow depression, tingling sensations, bloody urine, bloody stools, convulsions.

Comment: A sulfonamide derivative that can lead to kidney stones and hemolytic anemia.

Diupres (chlorothiazide plus reserpine)—See Diuril and Serpasil.

Diuril (chlorothiazide)—Diuretic, antihypertensive.

Adverse effects: Exacerbation or activation of lupus erythematosus, vomiting, cramping, diarrhea, headache, muscle spasms.

Comment: Particularly dangerous during pregnancy. Exposes both mother and fetus to unnecessary hazards. Does not prevent toxemia of pregnancy and is not valuable in treatment of that condition.

Elavil (amitriptyline)—Antidepressant, anxiety-reducing.

Adverse effects: Heart attacks, stroke, intestinal obstruction, delusions, excitement, numbness, incoordination, seizures, black tongue, breast enlargement, hair loss.

Comment: May increase psychotic symptoms and paranoia; may produce anxiety.

Enovid, Ovulen (norethynodrel with mestranol ethynodiol)—Prevention of pregnancy.

> *Adverse effects:* Blood clots, hypertension, stroke, heart attack, liver tumors, possible infertility, changes in sex drive.

> *Comment:* This is one of the few drugs that affects practically every organ system. The hazards that have been pinpointed in countless studies of oral contraceptives should make every woman think twice before taking them on a sustained basis. The hazards appear greatest for women who smoke.

Equanil, Miltown (meprobamate)—Anxiety, tension.

> *Adverse effects:* Slurred speech, congenital malformations, concentrates in breast milk, palpitations, fast pulse, aplastic anemia.

> *Comment:* Sustained use can lead to physical dependence, psychological dependence, and even fatal abuse.

Etrafon (perphenazine plus amytriptyline)—See Elavil and Trilafon.

Flagyl (metronidazole)—Trichomonas infections.

> *Adverse effects:* Incoordination, unpleasant taste, convulsions, depression, irritability, peripheral neuropathy (numbness and tingling), cystitis, decreased sex drive, EKG changes.

> *Comment:* Carcinogenic in experimental animals. Not to be used in pregnancy, when nursing, or with alcoholic beverages.

Haldol (haloperidol)—Major tranquilizer for psychotic disorders, Tourette's syndrome.

> *Adverse effects:* Fatal broncho-pneumonia, Parkinson-like syndrome, tardive dyskinesia (exaggerated muscular contortions), grande mal seizures, hallucinations.

> *Comment:* May cause irreversible brain damage when combined with lithium. Also interacts with alcohol, anticonvulsants, and anticoagulants.

Hydrodiuril (hydrochlorothiazide)—See Diuril.

Hydropres (hydrochlorothiazide plus reserpine)—See Hydrodiuril and Serpasil.

Hygroton (chlorthalidone)—Antihypertensive, diuretic.

Adverse effects: Weakness, lethargy, muscle fatigue, headache, yellow vision, aplastic anemia (bone marrow failure), hyperglycemia, impotence.

Comment: Make certain your doctor does blood studies periodically to detect electrolyte (blood chemical) imbalance.

Inderal (propranolol)—Hypertension, migraine, cardiac arrhythmia, angina.

Adverse effects: Congestive heart failure, tingling of hands, blood disorders, mental depression, catatonia, memory loss.

Comment: A potent drug often prescribed for hypertension, so dangerous that patients using it should be closely monitored. Among its numerous possible side effects is congestive heart failure. If a hypertensive patient dies while taking it, who can tell whether he died from the medicine or from the disease?

Indocin (indomethacin)—Arthritis.

Adverse effects: Perforation and hemorrhage of the esophagus, stomach, and small intestine—sometimes fatal; blurred vision, depersonalization, coma, deafness.

Comment: This drug is a hazardous analgesic that does not alter the progressive course of the disease. Its risks may dictate the choice of an alternative for the relief of pain.

Lasix (furosemide)—Diuretic, edema, hypertension.

Adverse effects: Ear noises, deafness, dry mouth, lethargy, jaundice, pancreatitis, blurred vision, anemia, urinary bladder spasm.

Comment: Not to be used during pregnancy or nursing; frequent blood tests should be performed. The drug is often prescribed for weight reduction, but is ineffective in reducing weight over the long term.

Librax (chlordiazepoxide plus clidinium)—Peptic ulcer (possibly effective).

Adverse effects: See Librium; also dry mouth, blurred vision, constipation, urinary hesitancy.

Comment: See Librium.

Librium (chlordiazepoxide)—Anxiety, tension.

Adverse effects: Drowsiness, confusion, changes in sex drive, jaundice, rage.

Comment: This drug's effectiveness after four months has never been established. Danger of physical and/or psychological dependence with extended use.

Limbitrol (chlordiazepoxide plus amytriptyline)—See Elavil and Librium.

Lithium (lithium)—Manic episodes and depression.

Adverse effects: Changes in kidneys, tremor, weakness, irreversible brain damage if used with Haldol, lack of coordination, blackout spells, incontinence, stupor, coma, circulatory collapse, thyroid abnormalities, EEG and EKG changes.

Comment: This is an old drug that has recently come back in vogue. The toxic dose is very near the therapeutic dose. It should not be given with diuretics.

Lomotil (diphenoxylate)—Diarrhea.

Adverse effects: Addiction, fast pulse, swollen gums, depression, headache, coma, toxic megacolon.

Comment: Related to the narcotic, Demerol. Interacts with barbiturates, alcohol, and tranquilizers.

Lopressor (metoprolol)—Hypertension.

Adverse effects: Tiredness, dizziness, depression, nightmares, insomnia, Peyronie's disease.

Comment: If given with digitalis and diuretics, heart failure may occur. May mask symptoms of hypoglycemia in diabetics.

Mellaril (thioridazine)—Psychotic disorders, depression, anxiety, agitation, sleep disturbances, fears, severe behavior problems in children, poor attention span, hyperactivity.

Adverse effects: Convulsions, loss of vision, orthostatic hypertension (more frequent in females), pseudo-parkinsonism, breast enlargement, edema, menstrual irregularities, false pregnancy tests.

Comment: This is another drug that produces some side effects that are identical with the symptoms it is supposed to relieve—confusion, hyperactivity, psychotic reactions, agitation.

Motrin (ibuprofen)—Arthritis.

Adverse effects: Peptic ulcers, gastrointestinal bleeding with fatal hemorrhage, visual disturbances, fluid retention, nervousness, ear noises, depression, insomnia.

Comment: Women should beware of this one, because antiarthritics are being promoted for the relief of menstrual cramps.

Mysoline (primidone)—Anticonvulsant.

Adverse effects: Birth defects in fetus, neonatal hemorrhage, vertigo, impotence.

Comment: Dangerous to give and dangerous to take away. Abrupt withdrawal may precipitate status epilepticus (prolonged seizures).

Naprosyn (naproxen)—See Motrin.

Parlodel (bromocryptine)—Suppress lactation, amenorrhea, galactorrhea (abnormal lactation).

Adverse effects: Headache, dizziness, fatigue, cramps, nasal congestion.

Comment: Acts on the pituitary gland, the master gland of the body; must have skull x-rays before using.

Pitocin (oxytocin)—Initiation or enhancement of uterine contractions.

Adverse effects: Tetanic uterine contractions, hypertension, brain hemorrhage, ruptured uterus leading to maternal and fetal deaths.

Comment: A powerful, dangerous drug that many obstetricians administer needlessly. Be sure the need to speed delivery is the health of mother and child, and not an appointment on the doctor's social calendar.

Pred-5, SK Prednisone, Aristocort, Kenalog, etc. (prednisone)—Endocrine disorders, rheumatic conditions, allergic states, etc.

Adverse effects: May mask signs of infection; cataracts, damage to optic nerve, hypoadrenalism in fetus, hypertension, chemical imbalance, psychic derangement, psychotic manifestations.

Comment: This is an adrenal cortical steroid that should be used selectively in the absence of less risky alternatives. Yet, it is one of the most overused drugs in modern medicine. It is even prescribed in topical preparations for treatment of minor skin conditions and may be absorbed and cause systematic effects.

Premarin (conjugated estrogens)—Vasomotor symptoms associated with menopause, atrophic vaginitis.

Adverse effects: Uterine cancer, damage to offspring, blood clots, liver tumors, high blood pressure.

Comment: The hazards associated with prolonged use of conjugated estrogens are so numerous that any woman taking them should question her doctor closely about potential secondary diseases resulting from their use. They have been reported in numerous studies to increase the risk of cancer. It would also be wise to read the cautions and warnings regarding use of this drug in the *Physician's Desk Reference,* which should be available in your local library.

Provera (medroxy-progesterone)—Some forms of abnormal uterine bleeding and some forms of failure to menstruate.

Adverse effects: Blood clots, loss of vision, double vision, migraine, acne, hirsutism, hair loss.

Comment: Increased risk of birth defects; affects virtually every organ system.

Raudixin (rauwolfia)—Antihypertensive, agitated psychotic states.

Adverse effects: Depression, nervousness, anxiety, nightmares, deafness, visual loss, arrhythmias, itching, impotence.

Comment: Contraindicated for patients with mental retardation. Drug-induced depression may persist for several months after drug is discontinued and may result in suicide.

Regroton (chlorthalidone plus reserpine)—See Hygroton and Serpasil.

Serapes (reserpine, hydrolazine, hydrochlorothiazide)—See Serpasil, Hydrodiuril, and Apresoline.

Serpasil (reserpine)—Hypertensive emergencies.

> *Adverse effects:* Angina-like symptoms, arrhythmias, slow pulse, anxiety, nightmares, parkinsonism, deafness, loss of vision, fainting, impotence, pseudolactation, water retention.
>
> *Comment:* Should be used only with extreme caution in patients with a history of mental depression, peptic ulcers, kidney damage, and patients on digitalis.

Sinequan (doxepin)—Psychoneurotic patients with depression or anxiety.

> *Adverse effects:* Increased symptoms of psychosis or shift to manic symptoms, fast pulse, hypertension, bone marrow depression, enlargement of breasts and milk secretion.
>
> *Comment:* Safety in pregnancy has not been established. Depressed patients should be closely monitored because of risk of suicide.

Stelazine (trifluoperazine)—Psychotic disorders, anxiety, tension.

> *Adverse effects:* Jaundice, bone marrow depression, increased angina, insomnia, amenorrhea, tardive dyskinesia, inhibition of ejaculation, cardiac arrest, impotence, sudden death.
>
> *Comment:* This drug affects the hypothalamus portion of the brain and may cause extrapyramidal effects such as muscle spasms, convulsions, difficulty in swallowing, and many other extreme effects. Study the prescribing information before taking the drug, so you will be alert to side effects that should be reported promptly to your doctor.

Tace (chlorotrianisene)—"Dry up" pills, menopausal vasomotor symptoms.

> *Adverse effects:* See Premarin; Enovid, Ovulen.
>
> *Comment:* As with other female sex hormones, a high price may be paid for the "benefit" of suppressing lactation.

Tagamet (cimetidine)—Duodenal ulcer.

Adverse effects: Muscle pain, dizziness, enlargement of the male breast, confusional states.

Comment: This is a relatively new drug which doctors, as usual, are hurrying to prescribe before widespread usage reveals additional adverse effects. Women hoping to conceive will be interested to know that the drug causes a drop in the sperm count of males who take it.

Tandearil (oxyphenbutazone)—Arthritis. See Butazolidin.

Thorazine (chlorpromazine)—Psychotic disorders, nausea, vomiting, manic-depressive illness.

Adverse effects: Nervous system depressant, jaundice, blood disorders, hypertension, EKG changes, psychotic symptoms.

Comment: May produce sudden death due to cardiac arrest and tardive dyskinesia, a severe muscular disorder that is sometimes irreversible.

Triavil (amytriptyline plus perphenazine)—See Elavil and Trilafon.

Trilafon (perphenazine)—Psychotic disorders, nausea, vomiting.

Adverse effects: Fever, arching of back, stiff neck, restlessness, tongue protrusion, slurred speech, parkinsonism, abnormal lactation.

Comment: Dangerous for patients with depression.

Tylenol/Codeine (acetaminophen and codeine phosphate)—Relief of mild to moderate pain.

Adverse effects: Liver damage, skin rash, itching, lowered blood sugar, disorientation, minor hallucinations, anemia, reduced sex drive or potency.

Comment: Prolonged use of codeine may lead to addiction. This drug is a respiratory depressant and should be used cautiously by persons with asthma or other breathing difficulties. Pregnant women should not take this drug.

Valium (diazepam)—Anxiety, tension, apprehension, fatigue, depressive symptoms, agitation.

Adverse effects: Drowsiness, fatigue, confusion, depression, jaundice, change in sex drive, anxiety.

Comment: This is the most overprescribed and probably the most abused drug in the United States. It may *produce* some of the symptoms it is supposed to relieve. In 1978 more than 1,500 persons—90 percent of them women—died in hospital emergency rooms from the misuse of tranquilizers such as Valium. Valium alone was responsible for an estimated 50,000 emergency room visits in 1978.

Vistaril (hydroxyzine)—Anxiety, tension associated with psychoneurosis, anxiety (prepartum and postpartum).

Adverse effects: Hypersedation, dry mouth, tremor, convulsions.

Comment: Because this drug is often used during labor, women should be aware that it may strengthen (potentiate) the action of Demerol and barbiturates by as much as 50 percent.

Zyloprim (allopurinol)—Gout, antiuric acid, kidney stones.

Adverse effects: Increase in attacks of gout early in treatment, hair loss, bone marrow depression, cataracts.

Comment: Skin rash may be followed by severe involvement of blood vessels, leading to liver damage and death.

Additional Reading

There are many excellent, thoughtful, carefully-researched books by women—most of them outside the medical profession—that explore individual aspects of medical mistreatment of women in greater depth. Among them are:

Arms, Suzanne. *Immaculate Deception: A New Look at Women and Childbirth in America.* Boston: Houghton Mifflin Company, 1975.

Brewer, Gail S., and Brewer, Tom, M.D. *What Every Pregnant Woman Should Know: The Truth about Diets and Pregnancy.* New York: Random House, 1977.

Corea, Gena. *Hidden Malpractice.* New York: William Morrow and Company, 1977.

Gordon, Barbara. *I'm Dancing As Fast As I Can.* New York: Harper & Row, 1979.

Haire, Doris. *The Cultural Warping of Childbirth.* Rochester, NY: International Childbirth Education Association, 1972.

Kilmartin, Angela. *Cystitis.* New York: Warner Books, 1980.

Lear, Martha Weinman. *Heartsounds.* New York: Simon & Shuster, 1979.

Scully, Diana. *Men Who Control Women's Health.* Boston: Houghton Mifflin Company, 1980.

Stewart, Lee, and Stewart, David, Ph.D. *Twenty-First Century Obstetrics Now.* Marble Hill, MO: NAPSAC, (P.O. Box 267, 63764), 1978.

My monthly subscription newsletter, *The People's Doctor Newsletter,* provides an ongoing source of authoritative documentation in matters affecting your health. $18 a year. Write P.O. Box 982, Evanston, IL 60204.

Index

213